NERV

All about the c nerves and
how they can be overcome with relaxation, improved
diet and exercise.

G000124332

THE NEW SELF HELP SERIES

NERVE TROUBLES

LEONARD MERVYN
B.Sc., Ph.D., C.Chem., F.R.S.C.

THORSONS

THORSONS PUBLISHING GROUP

First published in *The Science of Life* series
This edition published 1989

© THORSONS PUBLISHING GROUP 1989

*All rights reserved. No part of this book may be reproduced or utilized
in any form or by any means, electronic or mechanical, including
photocopying, recording or by any information storage and retrieval
system, without permission in writing from the Publisher.*

British Library Cataloguing in Publication Data

Mervyn, Leonard
Nerve troubles — 2nd ed.
1. Man, Nervous system. Therapy
I. Title II. Series
616.8'0468

ISBN 0-7225-2235-5

*Published by Thorsons Publishers Limited, Wellingborough,
Northamptonshire, NN8 2RQ, England*

Printed in Great Britain by Cox & Wyman Limited,
Reading, Berkshire

1 3 5 7 9 10 8 6 4 2

Contents

Note to reader

Before following the self-help advice given in this book readers are earnestly urged to give careful consideration to the nature of their particular health problem, and to consult a competent physician if in any doubt. This book should not be regarded as a substitute for professional medical treatment, and whilst every care is taken to ensure the accuracy of the content, the author and the publishers cannot accept legal responsibility for any problem arising out of the experimentation with the methods described.

1

Worry and Health

Nerve troubles are of two kinds, mental and physical. The first kind are caused by worry, and have to do with the mind rather than the body. The second kind are due to the systematic poisoning of the blood which nourishes the nerves. Both kinds, of course, are related. Worry can interfere with the proper digestion of food, and the resultant indigestion, lack of appetite and poor health will add to the person's worries. Conversely a constant nerve trouble, such as neuritis, will start a person worrying as to when and if it will pass, a factor which will tend to worsen the condition. So we see how the physical and the mental causes of nerve trouble react upon each other in a 'vicious circle'. Let us examine more closely the important relationship between worry and health.

This relationship between mind and body can give rise to psychosomatic illness when it is uncontrolled, and everyone will suffer at some time in their lives. What we feel or think is continuously having an effect upon our physical state. Mind and body have no clear-cut frontier between them.

Shock

Let us look at a common experience that has probably happened to all of us at some time. You have just avoided a nasty road or domestic accident that did you no physical harm, yet the prospect of what might have happened induces typical symptoms. You feel upset and physically ill, perhaps to such an extent that you are unable to continue what you were doing. If someone else is hurt, there is often a tendency to faint or vomit at the sight. Uncontrolled trembling and sweating of the palms often result. Your face looks pale and feels clammy, and your pulse beats faster than usual. Fainting combined with the other symptoms mentioned is popularly referred to as shock. Yet no physical harm has befallen you.

Shock is an acute condition brought on by the mind when it imagines what might have happened in a critical situation. Happily, it is usually only temporary but it demonstrates clearly how profoundly our bodily equilibrium can be upset by an emotional disturbance. Once the symptoms of shock, have passed, which may be as little as twenty-four hours later, it is easy to forget all about them. It is as well to remember them, however, because it is important to realize what shock can do to people when it happens to someone else. Try to bear this in mind next time you are tempted to tell someone that his sufferings are all imaginary. Occasionally, of course, shock and its after-effects are longer-lasting; in this case, professional help and sympathy are of paramount importance.

Effect upon the Digestive System

Through the inter-relation between mind and nervous system, the state of mental pandemonium known as worry has an immediate and powerful effect upon the digestion. The first thing that happens is that the gastric juice ceases to flow in any appreciable quantity. Then the peristalsis or rhythmic movements of the stomach, which mix the food mass and the gastric juice together very thoroughly, is interfered with. Thus, the mass of food is not mixed together properly and is also deprived of the digestive fluids and so it cannot be digested efficiently.

Medical literature abounds with examples where psychosomatic illness, associated with times of worry and stress, causes nervous indigestion. Individuals can develop persistent stomach pains with severe retching and vomiting when confronted by unpleasant situations or even other people they dislike. Jealous, over-protective or nagging parents and spouses can unwittingly cause such symptoms in their loved ones. Stress, too, is notorious for inducing gastric disorders. An example which proves this is the unusually high number of people with gastric ulcers whose condition became worse during the darker days of the Second World War.

Undigested Food becomes Poison

Worry, and similar mental states, such as fear, anger, excitement, resentment, frustration, anxiety, sorrow, and so on, causes indigestion with putrefaction of the contents of the stomach and intestines. In the course of this putrefaction various poisons known as toxins are produced. These poisons are then absorbed into the blood and carried to every tissue and organ. The disturbances resulting from this absorption of poisons, known as 'auto-intoxication', range from slight headache, dizziness or palpitation, to sudden death from 'heart failure' or 'apoplexy'. Stomach upsets, attacks of diarrhoea, and stomach and duodenal ulcers are all examples of what can happen when there is a regular build-up of these toxins.

Worry and the Heart's Action

So much for the effects of worry upon digestion and assimilation. There is another organ, however, upon which the influence of worry is even more disastrous. That organ is the heart, the regulator of the circulating blood. The nerve supply of the heart is peculiar. It consists of two sets of nerves known as the 'propulsive', which causes the heart to beat, and the 'inhibitory', which prevents the heart from beating too rapidly. When you are feeling calm, these two sets of nerves just balance each other, and your heart beats normally. If you become worried or frightened, however, the balance of this nervous apparatus is disturbed, and the rate of the heartbeat or pulsation is increased by between five and twenty beats a minute.

The Work of the Heart

The heart normally makes about seventy beats per minute. At every beat it propels a quarter pound of blood. The work it does in one day is equivalent to lifting 12.5 tons a distance of 1 foot. By adding ten extra beats per minute to the regular heartbeat, we increase the required work by the heart by about 2.5 tons. Therefore, if you are worried, the work your heart does is equivalent to raising about 15 tons a distance of 1 foot. The heart is a muscle, and this kind of over-exertion, particularly if it continues for months, or even years, often causes it to become abnormally developed, producing the disorder known as cardiac hypertrophy. Less commonly, the heart may actually be ruptured by some sudden mental or physical strain.

Worry and Blood-Pressure

The physical expression of an emotional upset may involve

any of the body systems. When the normal functions are upset or disordered by emotion, the illnesses that result are known as functional because no physical change has taken place in the body's structure, but the mechanism is not working properly. Such disorders are often temporary, but they can sometimes persist. If they go on for long enough, actual physical changes may occur in the organs affected. A temporary functional illness may clear up without any permanent ill-effects but once it becomes a physical organic business it will not always completely resolve. In such instances a scar, mental or otherwise, or some other permanent impairment of the organ or system will be left.

The most common side-effect of stress is a transient increase in blood-pressure. For a long time (usually several years), the sufferer's blood-pressure increases during stressful periods but reverts to normal between such periods. However, since an increase in blood-pressure is induced by changes in the blood vessel walls, a stage is eventually reached where the ability to revert to normal is weakened. The result is a permanent rise in blood-pressure. This tendency to develop high blood-pressure appears to be related more to those with the inability to express feelings of resentment and aggression. We tend to think that the person who is forever 'blowing his top' is the one most likely to develop high blood-pressure. 'Watch your blood-pressure!' we say to him. It now looks, though, as though blowing off steam is a good way to release pent-up tensions in a person.

Since blood-pressure is easily measured, it is an excellent indicator of how emotion or stress can affect an individual. It is one of the criteria used in the so-called lie detector tests. In the same way, even talking about emotional problems can cause transient increases in blood-pressure in sensitive people.

One classical case on medical record is a man who consistently sought his doctor's advice because of persistent upsets induced by an obnoxious relative. His blood-pressure was raised to such an extent that permanent hypertension was feared. Once the connection between emotion and blood-pressure was confirmed, the man overcame his problem simply by ignoring the snide and sarcastic remarks of his relative and severing all connections. His blood-pressure dropped immediately and has remained normal ever since. Anyone with a similar problem can try to tackle it in the same way, by diagnosing the cause and if possible removing it.

Medical confirmation of transient increases in blood-pressure for emotional reasons has come from observations on patients who already suffered from high blood-pressure. Their blood-pressure rose higher when discussing worrying personal affairs than when they were undergoing physical exercise. There is truth in the popular saying that 'it isn't work that kills, it's the worry'.

Worry is Mental Apathy

Worry is not suspense. Worry is not just anxiety, nor regret, nor fear, nor doubt, nor resolve. All these are mental and emotional states. Worry is essentially different from any of them. Worry is that vague, chaotic condition—that anarchy of the mind—in which hopes, fears, resolves, doubts, anxieties, regrets, anticipations and suspicions are all admitted to the mind. They constitute a ravening, destroying horde, under the influence of which logical reasoning is impossible, initiative is paralysed and the stability of the mind is threatened, and even destroyed. It should be clearly understood that the man or woman who yields to the habit of worry is not only certain to ruin health and personal efficiency, but is also in danger of losing his or her sanity. Worry is the most frequent cause of insanity.

Worry is a Curable Disease

Worry is a disease which is curable; but he who would be cured of it must cure himself. He must work out his own salvation. He must engage in a civil war of the intellect, and must reduce mental anarchy to mental order. He must, in other words, achieve self-control. And how is this to be accomplished? First, he must come to a full understanding of the fact that worry is never of the slightest use; indeed, since it prevents anything like clear thinking or firm resolution, it really makes matters worse. No one can think or decide on a course of action when he is worried. So he must resolve, no matter how bad matters seem to be, to face them quietly, calmly, thoughtfully, to plan as logically as possible, to act firmly and decisively, and then let results work themselves out. Most of the things we worry about never happen.

2

Stress

During the past thirty years, doctors and other health professionals have come to realize how heavy a toll stress is taking on our nation's well-being. In the United States of America, for instance, the American Academy of Family Physicians have calculated that two-thirds of consultations to general practitioners are prompted by stress-related symptoms. Leaders of industry have become alarmed by the vast costs of such symptoms in terms of absenteeism, lost productivity and medical recompense. The National Health Service in Britain counts such costs in terms of hundreds of millions of pounds in health benefits and medical expenses.

Stress is now known to be a major contributor, directly or indirectly, to coronary heart-disease, cancer, lung ailments, accidental injuries, cirrhosis of the liver, and suicide. These are amongst the ten leading causes of death in the western world. At the same time, stress is believed to play a role in aggravating such diverse conditions as multiple sclerosis, diabetes, genital herpes, and mouth and stomach ulcers. These complaints are reflected in the fact that the best-selling drugs in this and other countries of the western world are for treating gastric ulcers, high blood-pressure and depression (including tranquillizers). Dr Joel Elkes, a leading doctor of the University of Louisville, states 'Our mode of life itself, the way we live, is emerging as today's principle cause of illness'. Infection, once the prime killer, has now been conquered, only to be replaced by fatal diseases induced by our style of living.

The 'Fight or Flight' Reaction

Stress is not new. Prehistoric man, emerging from his cave after sleep, hears a rustling in the forest. His muscles tense, his heart pounds, his breath comes quickly as he faces some ferocious animal. The adrenaline flows as a result of his 'fight or flight' reaction. He decides to fight, picks up a weapon and chases off the animal. As it leaves, his body goes limp, his heartbeat reverts to normal and his breathing eases. The stress crisis is over and he starts again to work for survival for another day.

Modern man has changed little. He is not likely to meet fierce animals, but his day may start with a plunge into the chaos of rush-hour. He picks his way through traffic which is busy enough to make him late for work. He knows he is going to be late for that important appointment or unfinished report, so other stress factors are introduced. An unsympathetic boss suggests he should work late or forego his weekend to make up for lost time, and our unfortunate man feels he has reached the end. He would like to take the paperweight off his desk and fling it through that hated glass door, but he doesn't. Instead he sits down, his stomach churns, his back and neck muscles knot and, unbeknown to him, his blood-pressure starts rising. These are his responses to stress. His remedy is a tranquillizing tablet, a cigarette or a very strong alcoholic drink. Like his ancestor, his adrenaline flows, but for him there is no 'fight or flight' reaction. This would be quite impracticable. However, the same hormone can still cause changes so that his body responds as nature intended though the actions are repressed.

No one knows if there is more stress now than in earlier times, but many experts believe it has become more pervasive. We live in a world of uncertainties ranging from fear of losing a job to the lacing of our foods with unnatural additives and our bodies with unnatural medicines. Attempts to overcome stress vary from simple athletic pursuits like jogging to massaging over-taut muscles to a growing interest in hobbies far removed from our bread-winning jobs. As we shall see later in the book, all of us can also overcome the effects of stress, or more importantly prevent their happening in the first place, by careful selection of diets or supplementation with specific micro-nutrients. But first let us look a little further into the causes of stress and how the body's reactions to it can eventually induce harmful effects.

Causes of Stress Today

The upheaval in society's most basic values adds greatly to the general level of anxiety. A nationwide poll of more than 1000 married people aged 18 to 60 found that their greatest source of stress was the changes in society's attitudes towards sex, including sexual permissiveness and the new social roles of the sexes. Stress once took the form of an occasional calamity but is now regarded as a chronic relentless psychosocial situation, according to Dr Paul Rosch, director of the American Institute of Stress. Often the pressures of stress create thrill-seekers who find they prefer excitement to tranquillity and in so doing endanger their lives. They have become addicted to their own adrenaline secretions.

There is no adequate definition for the concept of stress. However the late Dr Hans Selye, the Austrian-born founding father of stress research, defined the condition as simply 'the rate of wear and tear in the body'. Others disagree and prefer to use the term to refer to any external stimulus that causes wear and tear or to the resulting internal damage. Little wonder there is confusion, and this is not helped by a more recent explanation: 'Stress, in addition to being itself, and the result of itself, is also the cause of itself, illogical though it may appear.'

Medical interest in stress began on the battlefield. In early conflicts, palpitations were so common that the condition was originally known as 'soldier's heart'. During the First World War, the complaint was called shell-shock, a crippling anxiety incorrectly attributed to damaged blood vessels in the brain. In the Second World War, the complaint was more sympathetically accepted and known as battle fatigue. It was during the aftermath of this conflict that Hans Selye and others proved that psychological strain or stress could cause dramatic hormone changes and hence clinical symptoms. Selye showed that when the 'fight or flight' response becomes long-lasting as it does in battle or other prolonged stress situations, long-term chemical changes occur, leading to high blood-pressure, an increased rate of hardening of the arteries, a lowered resistance to infection and many other problems.

Human beings have an annoying capacity to withstand massive doses of stress, according to Dr Fred Goodwin, director of the National Institute of Mental Health. Differences occur in our ability to mobilize our resistance to recurrent stressful episodes. The fact that nutrition can be one factor in determining our ability to withstand stress was observed and reported by Dr James Lind, a Scottish naval doctor, in the mid-eighteenth century. Dr Lind is accredited with the first published controlled clinical trial to determine how to prevent and cure scurvy. He proved that citrus fruits were effective but one important observation he reported was ignored at the time. Dr Lind noted that sailors under stress were the first to develop scurvy, despite eating the same diets as their fellows. In other words, the condition of stress induced a greater requirement for vitamin C or perhaps caused the vitamin to be used up at a greater rate. Dr Lind was not aware of the existence of vitamin C as such but his astute observation can now be explained in terms of what we know of the vitamin.

Researches into Stress

There was a great surge of research into stress in the early 1950s when the single common denominator was determined as 'the necessity for significant change in the life pattern of the individual'. It was found, for example, that amongst tuberculosis patients the onset of the disease generally followed a cluster of disruptive events such as a death in the family, a new job, change of house, or even marriage. Stress did not cause the illness, the tubercle bacillus did, but tension did promote the disease process.

It is even possible to measure the impact upon health of 'life-change events'. A Holmes-Rahe scale, based on studies of 5000 people in the 1940s and 1950s, attempted to rate the amount of social readjustments required for various events. At the top of the scale is death of a spouse (100 stress points), followed by divorce (73), marital separation (65), imprisonment (63) and death of a close relative (63). Not all stressful events are unpleasant; for example, marriage (50), pregnancy (40), buying a house (31) and Christmas (12).

A quantitative assessment of stress points was even more revealing amongst members of the medical profession. In a sample of eighty-eight young doctors, those with 300 or more stress points had a 70 per cent chance of suffering peptic ulcers, psychiatric disturbances, broken bones, heart problems and alcoholism. Those doctors who scored less than 200 stress points had only a 37 per cent incidence of these infirmities.

The impact of major life events on health is now generally accepted. A recent study in the *Lancet* (1983) reported that the incidence of fatal heart attacks rose sharply in Athens during the days following the 1981 earthquake there. High stress counts are linked to raised levels of the hormones associated with stress, particularly adrenaline, noradrenaline and endorphins. In Australia, a study has shown that eight weeks after the death of a spouse, widows and widowers have diminished immune responses which means they become more vulnerable to infection and cancer.

Everyday Annoyances

It now looks, though, as if stress is not necessarily associated with major life changes. There is a strong body of opinion, backed by excellent studies, that everyday annoyances of life, or 'hassles', contribute more to illness and depression than major life changes. Known as the 'snapped-shoelace factor', such minor annoyances include 'red-tape' in bureaucracy, paperwork in judiciary procedures, shift-work, work schedule changes, and excessive noise from traffic or airports. All these have been found to contribute to increased incidence of peptic ulcers, high blood-pressure, heart-disease and suicide.

Whether a single major change or a combination of trivial annoyances induce stress is less important than the consequences that one should be aware of. Divorce, for example, is not a single isolated event but can result in social isolation, a reduction in income and sometimes the problems of becoming a single parent. These then become the chronic stresses of life.

Loss of a job has a 'knock-on' effect—not the actual loss but rather the gradual domestic and psychological changes it imposes. Studies over twenty-five years indicate that for each 1 per cent increase in the national unemployment rate, there are 1.9 per cent more deaths from heart-disease; 2 per cent more from cirrhosis of the liver; 4.1 per cent more suicides; and an increase in mental health problems of 4.3 per cent for men and 2.3 per cent for women.

The fact remains, however, that not everyone falls to pieces or succumbs to a serious disease when they lose their spouse or job. The reasons that some cope better than others are manifold but some of the more important are related to nutrition and are dealt with later in the book. Diet and supplementation are not the whole story, of course, but self-help in other forms will also bring benefit. Recent studies indicate that help comes from the sense of being in control of one's life, having a network of friends or family to provide 'social support', and flexibility and hopefulness. Cancer, mental illness and suicides were found to be more related to lack of closeness to parents and a negative attitude towards one's family in almost 1400 medical students. The conclusion from this and other studies was that close relationships to others, either through family, friends or self-help groups, were the greatest and most reliable single contribution against stress that could not be tackled by other, including dietary, means.

The Effect of Work

Animals who can regulate stressful stimuli are better able to withstand the effects of stress. Being in control appears to make this difference, according to current research. Similarly, people who have little control over their jobs, such as cooks, assembly-line workers, garment makers and piecework labourers, in general have higher rates of heart-disease than those who can dictate the pace and style of their work. Worst off are waiters, telephone operators, cashiers and others whose work makes high psychological demands with little opportunity for independent decision-making. This combination of high demands and low control raises the risk of heart-disease as much as does smoking or having a high blood cholesterol level.

Two Stress Groups

Two main types of individual are now recognized amongst the general population as far as resistance to stress is concerned. Type A has a greatly increased susceptibility to heart attacks and other stress-related illnesses. Type A behaviour has two main components—first, there is the tendency to try to accomplish too many things in too little time; second, there is free-floating hostility. Such people are irritated by trivial things and exhibit signs of struggle against time and other people. Calmer individuals are classified as type Bs.

Many studies have shown that types A and types B respond differently to stress. In a typical example, hundreds of students were asked to perform a mental arithmetic task. The type A students produced forty times as much steroid stress hormone (cortisone) and four times as much adrenaline in their bodies as those of type B. The flow of blood to the muscles of type A was three times as great as that in type B. These differences had no effect upon the level of performance. Dr Redford Williams of Duke University in the USA, who carried out the study, concluded that the type A man was responding as though he were in an emergency or threatening situation. The increased secretion of cortisone and adrenaline would cause more fat to be released into the blood, and this could later be deposited around the heart. Little wonder, then, that persistently increased levels of these hormones might lead eventually to the inevitable stress-related diseases.

Type A individuals can help themselves in a number of ways, including modifying the diet, stopping smoking, losing weight, reducing salt intakes, cutting down on coffee (because of its caffeine content), taking holidays regularly, and indulging in some exercise. One effective measure is known as therapeutic relaxation or meditation. This practice can decrease heart rate, lower blood-pressure and reduce oxygen consumption by the muscles. It is essentially the exact opposite of the 'fight or flight' response. The supporters of therapeutic relaxation claim that the technique practised for ten to twenty minutes once or twice a day will produce a lasting reduction in high blood-pressure and other stress-related symptoms. It is a natural antidote to stress.

A relaxation response can also be achieved by following four simple steps: (1) assume a comfortable position; (2) close your eyes; (3) concentrate on a single word, sound or phrase; and (4) cast out all other thoughts. Taken together with related techniques like steady rhythmic breathing, self-hypnosis and muscle relaxation, such approaches are now beginning to be used to treat such stress-related problems as migraine, tension headaches, Raynaud's disease (constriction of the blood supply to the hands and feet), gastric ulcers, and colitis.

Similar approaches used under professional guidance have even succeeded in assuaging the anguish of cancer patients over the uncertainty of their future and the horrors of chemotherapy. The technique does not produce a cure but the cancer patient enjoys a happier lifestyle with the positive feeling of being in control of his life again. He can even be persuaded to imagine his tumour cells being destroyed by his own naturally-produced defender cells. This bizarre technique has helped many terminally-ill cancer patients but the benefits defy rational explanation in scientific terms. It is yet another example of the mysterious 'mind over matter' positive response to serious illness.

We shall see later how stress situations can also respond to specific dietary measures including high potency vitamin and mineral supplementation. First, however, we should consider some of the more common nerve troubles likely to be encountered in our everyday lives.

3

Nerve Problems

Before we examine what nerve disturbances can do to you and how they may be caused, let us look at how the nervous system is organized. It should be regarded as a vast network of cells which carry information in the form of nerve impulses to and from all parts of the body in order to bring about bodily activity.

A nerve impulse is defined as the electrical activity in the membrane of a nerve cell (also called a neurone) that by rapid spread from one region of the body to the next is the means by which information is transmitted throughout the nervous system. Impulses are carried along nerve fibres just as an electric current flows through a wire. Under resting conditions, a nerve is electrically charged because of different concentrations of certain minerals (notably calcium, magnesium, sodium and potassium) inside and outside the nerve cell. When an impulse is triggered, these minerals change places and in so doing allow the impulse to be propelled forward to the next nerve cell and so on. Once the cell has passed on its impulse, the minerals change places again to revert to their natural resting positions (that is, inside or outside the nerve) where they await the next impulse.

We shall see later how important it is for these minerals to be in the right proportions inside and outside nerve cells. If they are not, certain nervous problems arise because impulse propulsion is not uniform. Such abnormalities will only be cured by redressing the mineral balance, usually by overcoming dietary deficiencies of those minerals either with diet or supplementation.

The Nervous System

The nervous system is composed of:

1. The central nervous system formed from the brain and spinal cord. It controls the voluntary muscles and is responsible for the functioning of the special sense organs such as the eyes, as well as all movement and sensation in skin, muscles, bones and joints.

    The central nervous system is also in charge of all voluntary movement and action, such as walking, talking, singing, and so on. It is also the seat of the higher mental powers, such as reasoning, will-power, consciousness, memory, and emotion.

2. The remaining nervous tissue is known as the peripheral nervous system. This applies to all parts of the nervous system lying outside the brain and spinal cord. It includes the cranial nerves that arise directly from the brain and leave the skull through separate apertures, as well as the spinal nerves and their branches. These spinal nerves comprise thirty-one pairs that leave the spinal cord and are distributed to all parts of the body, passing out from the vertebral canal through the spaces between the arches of the spinal vertebrae. Each nerve pair has two bundles of nerves (called roots), one of which carries impulses

that cause movement. The other carries only impulses that cause the feeling of sensation. Once the roots have left the spinal cord, they immediately merge to form a mixed spinal nerve on each side. The spinal cord should therefore be regarded as the distribution centre that determines where nerve impulses concerned with both stimulation of movement and the senses will go.

The peripheral nervous system also includes the autonomic nervous system, which is responsible for the control of bodily functions that are not consciously directed. These include regular beating of the heart, intestinal movements, sweating, salivation, and even wound healing. We do not tell our lungs to breathe, our hearts to beat, our digestive systems to start, but they carry on even when we are asleep or unconscious. Muscles that are not directly under our conscious control are known as smooth muscles and are different in structure from those of our limbs, for example, which we can move at will.

The autonomic nervous system is subdivided further into sympathetic and parasympathetic nervous systems. Sympathetic nerves lead from the middle section of the spinal cord; parasympathetic nerves lead from the brain and lower spinal cord. The heart, smooth muscle and most glands receive fibres of both kinds. The reason for two sets of nerves is that they are antagonistic to each other so that their balance decides the functioning of the various organs they control. They do this by secreting from the nerve endings different chemical substances called neurotransmitters.

Sympathetic nerve endings liberate noradrenaline; parasympathetic nerve endings release acetylcholine.

Noradrenaline is a hormone that causes constriction of small blood vessels, leading to increased blood-pressure; increased blood flow through the arteries supplying the heart; a slowing of the heart rate; an increase in the rate and depth of breathing; and relaxation of the smooth muscle of the intestinal walls. Acetylcholine has actions essentially opposite to those of noradrenaline. At the same time it also increases the flow of tears, saliva and gastro-intestinal secretions.

The control and synthesis of both sets of neurotransmitters are partially under the influence of certain vitamins, minerals and other nutrients, which explains the importance of diet in maintaining a normal, healthy nervous system. These will be discussed later in the appropriate sections of the book.

To sum up, the autonomic nervous system controls all involuntary processes such as breathing, digestion, the pulsation of the heart, growth of hair and nails, healing of wounds, and vital functions generally. Without the central nervous system, man would possess no special sense organs such as sight and hearing. He would be like a vegetable, unable to move or feel. It is the central nervous system which puts us into touch with the world around us and provides us with all our experiences. The two systems, the central nervous system and the autonomic nervous system, are intimately linked, and along them nerve impulses are conducted to every part of the body. These nerve impulses move at the rate of 98 feet per second, varying with the temperature of the nerve fibre and other factors. Of the real nature of the nerve impulse, however, science can only speculate.

Let us now consider some of the more common nerve

problems most of which are disorders of the peripheral nervous system.

NEURALGIA

This is a term used to describe a severe burning or stabbing pain along a nerve or its branches. There are three types:

1. Trigeminal neuralgia (tic douloureux), characterized by brief paroxysms of searing pain felt along the distribution of one or more branches of the trigeminal nerve in the face.
2. Migrainous neuralgia, which is an acute facial pain lasting from thirty to sixty minutes and occurring at roughly the same time on successive days.
3. Post-herpetic neuralgia, an intense debilitating pain felt at the site of a previous attack of shingles.

Even when there is no dental trouble, it may feel as though all the teeth on one side of the jaw are aching.

The sufferer usually turns to 'pain-killers' containing aspirin, paracetamol, caffeine or codeine, and it is possible these may give him some temporary relief. The use of such drugs, however, cannot possibly effect a cure. In fact, they often prolong the trouble and make it worse by robbing the body of its vitamins and minerals. Neuralgia is an inflammation of the nerves and is frequently due to a deficiency of B-complex vitamins. It is closely related to the condition known as neuritis and mostly yields to treatment which aims at making good the vitamin deficiencies referred to.

Trigeminal Neuralgia

Trigeminal neuralgia or tic douloureux is so painful that the sufferer may be completely incapacitated. An attack of sharp, stabbing nerve pain in the face comes on without warning and may recur frequently or last for hours, and even days. Patients describe certain hypersensitive areas around the nose and mouth which when touched can trigger off an attack. Attacks can also follow exposure to cold, washing the face, talking, eating, or drinking. The cause of the complaint is unknown and no medical reasons can be found. Most sufferers are over 50 years of age, and females are affected more than males. It is estimated that there are upwards of one million sufferers from this ailment in the USA. The cause of tic douloureux is seldom revealed by orthodox methods and the usual treatment is to deaden the pain with powerful drugs.

The trigeminal nerve is the largest cranial nerve and as the name implies it splits into three divisions. The ophthalmic branch supplies sensory nerve fibres to the eyeball, eyelids and tear glands. In addition, some find their way to the nose and the skin of the brows and scalp. The second branch is the maxillary nerve which supplies stimulatory fibres responsible for controlling the muscles involved in chewing; the sensory nerves relay information about temperature, pain and touch from the whole front half of the head, including the mouth. The third branch, the mandibular nerve, controls the senses and responses of the lower jawbone.

It is therefore not difficult to see how any abnormality of the trigeminal nerve can cause pain in any part of the face. In trigeminal neuralgia it is not always the part that is touched that causes the excruciating pain. The distribution of the nerve branches are such that any part of the head can be the trigger to cause pain anywhere in the area of the face.

Though the cause of trigeminal neuralgia is not known, some interesting theories have been put forward over the years. One theory about tic douloureux and its treatment has been advanced by W. J. Hanes, M.D., allergy specialist at Bryn Mawr Hospital in Pennsylvania, USA. Dr Hanes discovered that some patients suffering from tic douloureux obtained relief after he had administered antihistamine for allergy ailments from which they also suffered. But he found that, while antihistamines brought a measure of relief, the most valuable treatment was the oral administration of hydrochloric (stomach) acid whose principal function is the digestion of proteins. A further discovery was that milk was a contributing factor to this agonizing type of neuralgia. In 220 cases of tic douloureux that he treated, the oral administration of hydrochloric acid brought complete relief in 131 cases or just a little below 60 per cent of all cases, while partial relief was experienced by 23 patients (10.4 per cent) so that in all 70 per cent of the patients benefited. These results and subsequent studies by Dr Hanes suggested that tic douloureux could arise from a deficiency of hydrochloric acid in certain persons. This deficiency might arise in turn because of the ageing process. As a body ages, the secretion of hydrochloric acid tends to diminish. Studies made by the well known Mayo Clinic in the USA of 3746 medical histories revealed that both sexes showed a decline in the secretion of stomach acid after the age of 40 and that from 50 years onwards the deficiency became progressively more marked.

Milk Should be Avoided
Another cause for lack of stomach acid is excessive milk consumption. Milk neutralizes stomach acid. This is why medical men prescribe plenty of milk for patients with stomach ulcers. Dr Hanes considers that sufferers from tic

douloureux should omit milk from their diet. Milk has large protein molecules which, if not reduced by stomach acid, are not completely assimilated. Partially undigested protein molecules then enter the blood. The blood regards them as foreign invaders, and manufactures antibodies to destroy them. Unfortunately, one of the by-products of this manufacturing process is histamine which gives rise to various allergy reactions, of which a form of cold in the head (allergic rhinitis) and asthma are common examples. Milk is now becoming recognized as a prime stimulator of allergies. It is also mucus forming and should be viewed with suspicion by all who suffer from an allergy as well as those subject to catarrh, sinusitis and other ailments of the respiratory system. We advise sufferers from tic douloureux to give Dr Hanes' ideas a trial by omitting milk from their diet, as well as milk products such as cheese and milk puddings, and to take a hydrochloric acid preparation daily.

Hydrochloric acid may be taken as a supplement in solid form as betaine hydrochloride and glutamic acid hydrochloride. Betaine hydrochloride provides 23.8mg hydrochloric acid per 100mg. The usual dose is 60-500mg taken as tablets with water which is drunk just after meals. Glutamic acid hydrochloride provides only 19.9mg hydrochloric acid in 100mg. The usual dose is 600-1800mg which should be taken with water and drunk after meals. It is reported that twenty-four physicians in various parts of the USA, Canada and Europe have used Dr Hanes' treatment for tic douloureux with good results.

Vitamin B$_1$ (thiamine)
According to Dr John Marks, a Fellow of the Royal Society of Medicine, in his book *A Guide to the Vitamins, their Role*

in Health and Disease (published by Medical and Technical Publishing Co. Ltd, St. Leonard's House, Lancaster, England, 1975), large doses of vitamin B_1 have been recommended to treat trigeminal neuralgia. He reports that he has seen success in such cases with daily intakes of between 50-600mg vitamin B_1, preferably taken divided into two or three doses.

Migrainous neuralgia

Although this may respond to some of the dangerous drugs used to treat migraine (see page 28), there are also natural approaches to its prevention and treatment in the medical literature. A similar daily dose of vitamin B_1 as that suggested for trigeminal neuralgia may help relieve the condition. Dr John Marks also reports that vitamin B_2 (riboflavin) taken at the rate of 10mg with each meal may also help.

Post-herpetic neuralgia (post-shingles neuralgia)

Shingles or herpes zoster is due to a viral infection that affects the nerve endings in the skin. It usually starts with pain along the distribution of a nerve, often in the face, chest or abdomen, followed by the development of small blisters. Although the disease subsides in about three weeks, severe pain caused by post-herpetic neuralgia may persist for many months in the affected area.

The most natural treatment of the neuralgia is a high potency vitamin B complex taken as soon as the original nerve pain occurs and continued through the whole period of the disease. Vitamin B_{12} is particularly useful in treating shingles but because this vitamin is only absorbed to a limited extent, intramuscular injections are needed to introduce high concentrations. Nevertheless, when taken orally along with other members of the B complex, vitamin B_{12} can give some relief from post-herpetic neuraliga. The best way, of course, is to prevent the condition arising in the first place by prompt therapy.

NERVE ROOT DISORDERS

Nerve root dysfunction generally follows pressure upon or invasion of a root. Nerve roots may also be involved in vitamin deficiency diseases like pernicious anaemia, producing a profound loss of sensation. The most likely nerve root disorder is produced by mechanical compression of the nerve by a herniated disc, commonly known as a slipped disc.

Slipped Disc

Pain is typical of nerve root complaints and it is often precipitated by movement of the spine. This is because the cartilaginous disc, which forms a strong buffer pad between the vertebrae, can slip out from between them leaving the nerve root compressed between the bones. Usually this occurs on one side or the other but if enough of the disc is displaced, the condition becomes bilateral and pain is felt on both sides of the area.

Pain in the area to which the compressed root is distributed may begin suddenly and severely but sometimes it is quite insidious. It is worse on movement and can be worsened by a simple action like coughing, laughing or straining (as in defaecation). The area of the spine affected determines where the pain will be.

If the pain is low down, raising the legs can cause pain in the back. If it is high up, simply flexing the neck causes an acute pain in the area. Muscles supplied by the impaired nerve root eventually become weak, wasted, flabby and lacking in firmness. There may be fasciculation, a brief

spontaneous contraction of a few muscle fibres, seen as a
flicker of movement under the skin.

Cervical Nerve Root Disorder

This is a nerve root condition affecting the seven bones that
make up the neck or cervical region of the backbone. The
great flexibility of this part of the spine predisposes it to acute
injury from sudden motion as in whiplash injury, usually
produced by a sudden jerk of the head backwards. This often
happens in motor accidents. Other causes include athletic
injuries, sudden pulls or thrusts on the arms, and falls.
Occasionally inflammation and infections are the cause.

As they get older, many people suffer low-grade
inflammation caused by wear and tear of the cartilage discs
between the cervical vertebrae. Eventually the nerve roots
become compressed as the space in which the nerves are
carried becomes constricted. The condition is often worsened
by continued motion of the neck vertebrae. This is why
immobilization of the neck in surgical collars is often the
first line of treatment in medicine.

When the cervical nerve roots are compressed, pain is the
most frequent complaint. Sometimes it is in the neck but
it can occur anywhere along the distribution of the neck
muscles. Pain most commonly radiates between the shoulder
blades and to the tops of the shoulders. In some people,
associated muscle contraction may cause pain to radiate into
the upper arms. Neck or shoulder motion, particularly neck
extension or tilting, may be limited. It may cause pain or
crunching sounds in the neck muscles; 'knots' may also be
present. Often nerve root involvement may be accompanied
by numbness and tingling in the skin and by sensory loss
in the hands.

Although the pain in these nerve root disorders is due to compression of the nerve, treatment of the condition is aimed at the inflammation or arthritic process causing the compression. Pain killers like aspirin will have both an analgesic and an anti-inflammatory effect and they are often the first line of treatment. However, as discussed later in the book, all drugs have some disadvantages.

Natural treatments for these disorders include herbal remedies (Devil's Claw), vitamins (B complex, particularly pantothenic acid and B_{12}) and extract of New Zealand green-lipped mussels. Dietary approaches, with the emphasis on alkaline-producing foods rather than acid-producing foods, have also been claimed to prevent and treat these conditions. Once the factor causing the nerve compression is controlled, relief of pain and cure usually follows.

NEURITIS or PERIPHERAL NEURITIS

This condition is also known as neuropathy or peripheral neuropathy. It is a disease of sensory, motor, reflex or blood vessel nerves that can affect one or more nerves. When a single nerve is affected, it is termed mononeuropathy or mononeuritis; two or more nerves affected in separate areas is mononeuritis multiplex; many nerves simultaneously affected give rise to the complaint of polyneuropathy, polyneuritis or multiple peripheral neuritis. The lesions are usually degenerative in nature and can occur in the nerve roots or peripheral nerves.

For our purposes, neuritis means an inflamed condition either of a single nerve or of two or more nerves in separate areas. It can be due to direct blows, penetrating injuries, contusions, compression, fracture or dislocation of bones. Violent muscular activity or over-extension of the joints can cause neuritis. People who grip small tools tightly or operate air hammers can be subject to neuritis. It can also arise from localized infections and from ingesting toxins such as lead, arsenic, mercury, or bismuth. It may also be caused by some drugs.

It should be clear that the nerves most frequently used will become most painful. Thus a tennis player may experience neuritis in the elbow and shoulder, a person who lifts heavy loads would feel pain in his back, a postman in his legs, a typist in the forearms, and so on. This type of neuritis is very common.

The most usual cause of neuritis is nutritional or metabolic. Almost always, a polyneuropathy can result from nutritional deficiency (especially of the B vitamins). This is usually caused by a poor diet, devitalized food, alcoholism, pernicious anaemia (where the vitamin B_{12} cannot be absorbed), drug-induced vitamin B_6 deficiency, malabsorption of vitamins, and psychoses (severe mental illnesses). Polyneuropathy also occurs in thyroid deficiency, some blood diseases and in patients with kidney disease receiving dialysis treatment. Several forms of neuropathy can occur in diabetes mellitus.

In severe cases such as these it is advisable to take two B-complex tablets and one vitamin B_1 (10mg) tablet three times daily before meals. Between meals, a dessertspoonful each of brewer's yeast powder and non-fat milk powder should be taken, mixed in a glass of water and sweetened (if needed) with a teaspoonful of honey. This drink is rich in B-complex vitamins, calcium, phosphorus, lactose, protein and iron. Sometimes even higher potencies of the B complex are required.

NEURASTHENIA

We live in a neurotic age, of wars and rumours of wars, of

depressions, of economic 'boom and bust', an age notorious for its rising incidence of debt and tax bondage, an age in which, in the short intervals of 'peace' between wars, the machine constantly displaces men from the employment system. Taken all in all, the frenzied age in which we live is notorious for its insecurity, its morbid fears, its doubtful happiness. In such an unstable world, it is small wonder that the nerves of many people are unhinged, and that they seek escape from their dark fears and great anxieties in such opiates as television, films, racecourses, clubs, and a frantic whirl of entertainment to keep their minds off the stark realities of life.

Neurasthenia is a set of psychological and physical symptoms (called a syndrome) including fatigue, irritability, headache, dizziness, anxiety, and intolerance of noise. It can be caused by organic damage such as head injury or, as we have seen above, by neurosis. It can be the outcome of a scheme of life noted for its wrong feeding, frenzied living and chaotic thinking.

It is a condition in which the whole nervous system has been systematically starved of the B and E vitamins by the refining of flour, a process which removes vitamins and minerals from grains to leave a demineralized, denatured 'foodless' food from which we make our daily bread. To treat the condition with one of the proprietary nerve tonics on the market, or with any tonic prescribed by a doctor, merely serves to dope the sufferer a bit, so that he may be less jumpy, less sensitive to his condition. Such treatment is not curative. In the long run, the poisonous nature of these drugs will accentuate the condition. Medical advisers also tell neurasthenics 'not to worry', to 'go away for a change', and so on. This is good advice so far as one is able to take it, but the exhortation of people 'not to worry' rarely, if ever, has the desired effect. The one thing that neurasthenics can't help doing is worry. Worry has become habitual with them. It is part of the complaint from which they suffer. To urge them 'not to worry' is therefore a rather idle counsel of perfection. However, as we shall see, a plan of attack on neurasthenia is laid down in this book. It usually works like a charm.

NERVOUS BREAKDOWN

A nervous breakdown (sometimes called nervous collapse) indicates that the nervous system has become exhausted. This implies that the fault is somewhere in our nervous organization, or the human computer which is that part of ourselves which knows who we are, what we want to do and how to go about it. Just as man-built computers can blow a fuse as a result of overloading, so the human mind can be put under too much stress and break down in a similar manner. The result is that the person grinds to a halt and cannot go on. If things really get out of hand, he or she weeps, rushes about, attacks himself (sometimes to the extent of attempted suicide) or attacks someone else. Most of us regard this as a nervous breakdown.

In the popular idiom, individuals will admit to having 'bad nerves', when they feel something is wrong resulting in an undesirable state of health. What they mean is that they are suffering from irritability, anxiety and some degree of depression. Often they will admit 'my nerves have gone', meaning the same thing.

When someone admits that he is 'a nervous person', this does not imply an illness of any sort but simply that he considers himself to be more sensitive and more easily upset than the next person. He compares himself with others who are more 'thick-skinned' and accepts that his personality is different. It is generally accepted, though not necessarily true, that this type of individual is more likely to have a nervous breakdown.

Most people imagine their nerves, by which they mean their central nervous system, to be similar to violin strings. Stretch them too far and they reach breaking point and snap—the result is a nervous breakdown. As far as they are concerned, the mind resides in the brain so that their awareness of themselves (the mind) and the anatomical nerves (the central nervous system) are one and the same thing. To the lay person, the condition of 'nerves' is a collective term for nervousness, irritability, anxiety and depression.

As far as these people, are concerned, a nervous breakdown is something that happens to a person and happens inside him or her. It implies that something serious has happened as a result of which the person is no longer functioning properly and hence is no longer responsible for his or her actions. The condition may arise from late hours, overwork, loss of sleep and emotional stress such as worry or grief.

What sort of people are likely to suffer a nervous breakdown? As we have seen, people with 'bad nerves' might if they do not seek help or attempt to help themselves. Anyone under stress is at a high risk and, as we have already seen in the previous chapter, stress can take many forms. Weak people (or those with hidden weakness) represent a vulnerable group, whether 'weak' is used in a physical, emotional or moral way. Because they are vulnerable, such individuals have fewer options or escape routes than others.

Cranks or eccentrics are often regarded as more susceptible to nervous breakdowns than 'normal' people. These individuals are often eccentric because they are more vulnerable or vice versa. Whatever the cause, their strongly-held or excessive beliefs protect them from the anxiety of uncertainty. Once these are challenged and their belief is destroyed, they have no other way to turn and the result is an extreme nervous breakdown.

This group is a minor one. At the other end of the scale are the people who live on their own or are isolated. More single and separated or divorced people are likely to end up with a nervous breakdown according to modern studies. Married life brings its own trials and tribulations but having someone to lean on, even if you don't like him or her, is better than having no one at all with whom to share your troubles.

Why should some people or sectors of the population be more likely to suffer a nervous breakdown than others? No one is quite sure but it is interesting to note that the people in the above-mentioned groups are also those who tend to be deficient in vitamins and minerals because of poor diets that have been denuded of essential micro-nutrients. Stress and any sort of excessive mental pressure on the nerves are both known to increase our requirements for vitamins and minerals. Little wonder then that diets that provide barely the minimum amounts of these nutrients will gradually induce an insidious deficiency in these individuals. Later we shall see how important adequate vitamins and minerals are in nourishing the nervous system. When its needs are increased and not met, nerve problems will certainly follow.

MULTIPLE SCLEROSIS

Formerly known as disseminated sclerosis, this condition is the most common of the so-called demyelinating diseases.

Myelin is the sheath that surrounds nerve fibres, rather like the insulating material that covers an electrical wire. Not all nerves are protected by a myelin sheath but those that are conduct nerve impulses more rapidly than those that are not. Myelin consists of a complex material made up of protein and lecithin, a phospholipid consisting of polyunsaturated fatty acids, phosphorus and choline. Cholesterol is also an important component of myelin.

The myelin sheath around the nerves of the brain and spinal cord can be damaged, which affects the function of the nerves involved. The body then exacerbates the damage by attempting to repair it but instead of laying down healthy sheath material in the damaged areas, it replaces them with hard connective tissue which cannot conduct nerve impulses. The result is a hardening or sclerosing of the myelin sheath and nerve which gives rise to the condition of multiple sclerosis.

Sometimes the myelin sheath is not even repaired and its structure then resembles an electric cable with worn insulation. The result is similar to the short circuit that is the inevitable result of poor insulation. We can replace a worn electric cable easily but a worn myelin sheath can only be replaced from inside the body itself.

Some people believe that demyelination giving rise to multiple sclerosis is due to a virus but the offending micro-organism has never been isolated. There is no specific medical treatment of the complaint but there is hope that, at least for some sufferers, diet and specific supplementation may play a role in slowing down the insidious development of the disease once it has been diagnosed.

Dietary approaches include exclusion diets; diets rich in polyunsaturated fatty acids; diets low in fats; diets high in protein; gluten-free diets; mineral and vitamin supplementation, and increased intakes of vegetable oils but in particular oil of evening primrose. The latter is based upon some evidence that an inability to heal damaged myelin is due to a lack of polyunsaturated fatty acids or loss of the means to convert dietary polyunsaturated fatty acids to the components of the phospholipid of the sheath.

Some believe that those suffering from multiple sclerosis are unable to convert linoleic acid (found in vegetable oils) into gamma linolenic acid (found in only a limited number of vegetable oils). This first step is absolutely essential in metabolizing dietary polyunsaturated fatty acids. By giving oil of evening primrose or other edible vegetable oils containing pre-formed gamma linolenic acid, the blockage in multiple sclerosis is bypassed.

All of these dietary measures and others are assessed critically in *Multiple Sclerosis, A Self-help Guide to its Management*, by Judy Graham, published by Thorsons.

4

Sleep, Pain and Drugs

The Importance of Sleep

Sleep is defined as 'the periodic state of rest in which there is diminution of consciousness and activity'. During sleep the heart slows down, the body temperature falls slightly, the breathing becomes slow and rhythmic and there is in some mysterious way a recharging of the body's batteries that have been depleted during daytime activities.

Sleep has several stages characterized by EEG patterns and related to eye movements. EEG are the initials for electroencephalogram, a tracing from a machine developed for recording the electrical activity from different parts of the brain. The pattern of the EEG reflects the state of the subject's brain and his level of consciousness in a characteristic manner. Hence it is a useful tool in studying the mechanics of sleep.

Periods of rapid eye movement (REM) are generally associated with dreaming and rapid activity is seen on the EEG. These periods occur five to six times during a normal night's sleep and accounts for 20-25 per cent of the total sleep-time. Sleep-inducing drugs affect EEG patterns and most tend to depress REM sleep. The lack of REM or dreaming time has not been demonstrated to have any adverse consequence in those taking these drugs. However, you should be warned that abrupt withdrawal of a REM-suppressive drug can result in a rebound increase (up to 45 per cent) in the amount of REM sleep, causing sleep disturbances, vivid dreams or nightmares.

The French say 'Who sleeps, dines'. Sleep does not take second place, even to food. Man can go without food for a month, but few can survive three or four consecutive sleepless nights. We sleep for a third of our lives, so sleep is evidently regarded by nature as important. No form of rest is so complete as sleep, which is often elusive, yet there are no rules on how to fall asleep. You cannot will yourself to sleep—it must be enticed. Shakespeare expressed this fact in *King Henry IV*:

> Sleep, O gentle sleep
> Nature's soft nurse, how have I frighted thee
> That thou no more wilt weight my eyelids down
> and steep my senses in oblivion.

There is much that scientists do not know about sleep, but they are aware that sleep mostly follows fatigue, a diminished blood supply to the brain, and a cessation of mental activity. They know, too, that the early hours of a sleep are the deepest and probably the most important.

Insomnia

Insomnia or the lack of ability to sleep can take at least four forms: an inability to fall asleep rapidly; frequent awakenings from sleep; early awakening with the inability to fall asleep again; and unrefreshing or non-restorative sleep. Sleep disturbance can be temporary, when a person has some anxiety or depression that interferes with sleep.

Poor sleepers can take a short walk or engage in light exercise before going to bed, to encourage fatigue. Some find that a warm bath, or a tepid shower and rub-down before bed will induce sleep, while others may need an unexciting book and to sip a glass of warm milk to encourage sleep. During sleep the brain tissue becomes anaemic and actually shrinks. After a hearty meal the digestive system draws blood from the brain to aid assimilation and a sleepy feeling often follows. An ample supply of blood to the brain favours mental activity and the converse is also true. This is why soaking one's feet in water for ten minutes before retiring helps sleep. The moist heat draws blood from the brain, discouraging thought processes. Sleep comes more easily and restfully before midnight than after it, and late hours usually bring in their train undue mental activity and sleeplessness.

The first approach of sleep is gentle and touches the mind lightly. This is the psychological moment to drop off, a process helped by being still and relaxed, and breathing slowly and rhythmically. The bedroom should be airy, dark and quiet, but a ticking clock seems to aid sleep. The body should be relaxed and comfortably warm, and the pillows not too high. Never retire with cold feet and don't take tea or coffee just before going to bed as both beverages contain caffeine, an alkaloid drug which stimulates mental activity. Avoid argument and contention before retiring, as they inflame the emotions and sleepless hours may elapse before the fire burns out.

Sleep and the Elderly

The belief that elderly people do not need as much sleep

as younger people is challenged in an article in the *Lancet*. Records kept of eighty-three active people over the age of 60 years who had no organic disease showed that more than half of those who slept less than seven hours complained of insomnia, whereas of those who slept eight hours or more, less than a third complained of any symptoms. The thirty-four patients who slept for less than seven hours were told to spend at least nine to ten hours in bed at night and to rest during the day. All these patients said they felt much better as a result.

Natural Sleep-Inducing Agents
Dr Carl C. Pfieffer, Director of Princeton's Brain Bio Center, uses the technique of electroencephalography (EEG traces) to study natural biochemical stimulants and sleep-inducing agents. His method allows the measurement of stimulants, sedatives, hypnotics and anti-psychotic drugs in man. In this way he can compare any substance with others in its action on the central nervous system.

When studying vitamins in his system, he found that thiamine (vitamin B_1) and ascorbic acid (vitamin C) have an anti-anxiety or sedative effect. A sedative is a substance that has a calming effect, relieving anxiety and tension. The effect of vitamin C, when given at a dose of 1000mg, lasted for a full six-hour test period. It was the most effective vitamin studied and is at present being followed up as an anti-anxiety agent useful in neuroses. Thiamine also has a useful action at the 100mg dose.

These were single doses tested under experimental conditions and each individual in practice may find that lower intakes taken on a regular daily basis can have a similar though more prolonged anti-anxiety effect.

The spinal cord nerves and brain contain high concentrations of the B vitamin inositol. The cerebrospinal fluid, the liquid that bathes the nerves of the spinal cord and the brain, is also rich in inositol, containing about four times the level in blood. Dr Pfieffer found that inositol is sedative and can be used to treat insomnia and anxiety problems. Whilst a good, balanced diet will contain about 1g of inositol, this amount is unlikely to be provided in the poor diets many people subsist on. Hence Dr Pfieffer recommends supplementary inositol at up to 1g morning and night to allay anxiety and help induce sleep.

Another natural sleep-inducing agent is pyridoxine (vitamin B_6). This vitamin is essential for the production of brain transmitter substances, amongst which is gamma aminobutyric acid (GABA). This is a natural calming agent that can induce natural sleep. When the vitamin is deficient, particularly in babies, the result is convulsions. The relationship of pyridoxine to sleep is also through its action in dream recall.

At the Brain Bio Center, they have discovered that dream recall can serve as a means of measuring brain-pyridoxine deficiency. Dream recall is simply the ability to recall dreams upon waking. Sometimes this may happen immediately but some people may recall their dreams at any time before the next sleep. When pyridoxine in the brain is deficient, dream recall is inefficient.

The amount of pyridoxine needed for normal dream recall, and the time at which it should be taken, is specific for each person. If, for example, too much pyridoxine is taken or it is taken with the evening meal, dreams become so vivid that the patient is awakened from sleep all night long. Such a restless-dream phenomenon is disturbing so the dose of pyridoxine should be reduced to that which induces normal sleep and dreaming patterns.

Dr Pfieffer reports that he himself needs 50mg pyridoxine each morning to sleep and dream normally at night whilst he is at work at the Brain Bio Center. When he takes this dose whilst on holiday (that is, during a less stressful period) he dreams excessively. On holiday, he therefore reduces his ideal dose to 25mg pyridoxine. Anyone who wishes to establish a normal sleep and dream pattern must find his own ideal dose. The lowest dose is the best and is preferably taken in the morning, presumably to allow time for the brain pyridoxine levels to build up.

Drugs for Nervous Conditions

Let us now look at the types of medicinal drugs used to treat the various nervous conditions described above. They are most conveniently divided into three groups; hypnotics, sedatives and tranquillizers.

Hypnotics and sedatives depress the central nervous system. Whilst hypnotics are used to induce sleep, sedatives relieve anxiety and restlessness in the waking person without inducing sleep. There is no sharp distinction between the two effects and often the same drug is used for both. The difference is in the dosage used and the method employed in giving the drug. A high dose of either may depress the nervous system sufficiently to produce a state of coma.

Normal sleep is composed of two alternating phases, a non-dreaming or slow wave (EEG) and rapid eye movement (REM) in which, as we have seen, most dreaming takes place. The non-dreaming phase is generally itself divided into four further stages varying from drowsiness to deep sleep.

Hypnotic drugs reduce the duration and intensity of REM

sleep. This is why when hypnotics are withdrawn there is often a rebound phenomenon and extra dreaming takes place. Changes in the brain after prolonged used of some hypnotics can produce tolerance to the drugs and it may take weeks or months for conditions to return to normal. Dependence is a particular feature of the barbiturate-type drugs but can occur with any of the sedatives and hypnotics. It is characterized by an increased need for the drug resulting in a tendency to take more and hence a mental and physical dependence on the effects of the drug. A vicious circle sets in which is difficult to break.

Two examples of commonly used hypnotics are the barbiturates and nitrazepam, a non-barbiturate. Whilst barbiturates differ tremendously in their dosage, in duration of action and in the margin of safety between therapeutic and toxic doses, all have several disadvantages. These include tolerance, liability to abuse, severe withdrawal effects, hangover effect, possibility of dependence, and an enhancement of their effect by alcohol. To these may be added drowsiness and lethargy and occasionally skin eruptions and gastro-intestinal disturbances. The elderly may experience restlessness, excitement and a worsening of the symptoms of the nervous disorders for which they are being treated.

Nitrazepam belongs to a group of drugs called benzodiazepines which are often preferred to barbiturates because they have a wider margin of safety. Despite this, it is known that prolonged use of nitrazepam may lead to dependence of the barbiturate type described above. In addition, the drug can cause drowsiness, hangover and light-headedness. Confusion has been reported in elderly people. Children given high doses may have excessive secretion of mucus and saliva. Because of the wider safety margin of nitrazepam and similar drugs, they are increasingly being prescribed in preference to the barbiturates when a hypnotic is required.

In addition to these hypnotic and sedative drugs, tranquillizers are widely used today in treating nervous diseases. The term tranquillizer denotes drugs which are capable of inducing a state of calm in an individual but do not induce hypnosis. Tranquillizers are classified into two groups—major and minor. The major type, which include the phenothiazines and lithium carbonate, are used mainly for the treatment of psychoses such as schizophrenia, mania, senile dementia and behaviour disorders in children.

Chlorpromazine is a typical major tranquillizer of the phenothiazine type. Its side-effects include drowsiness, dryness of the mouth, pallor of the skin, weakness, low body temperature, fast heartbeat, irregular pulse, agitation, insomnia, depression, and skin rashes. More seriously, jaundice and blood problems can be caused by the drug. Weight gain can also occur.

The so-called minor tranquillizers like diazepam, although regarded as perfectly safe in the past, are now beginning to exhibit serious side-effects. The mild and infrequent effects of drowsiness, light-headedness and ataxia (shaky movements and unsteady gait) have been known for some time. However, low blood-pressure, gastro-intestinal upsets, visual disturbances, skin rashes, urinary retention, headache, confusion, and vertigo have also been reported. Blood diseases and jaundice are occasional side-effects. More disturbing, however, is the finding that dependence or addiction of the barbiturate-type can be a property of the mild tranquillizers like diazepam. Convulsions can be induced in some people by sudden withdrawal of high doses of the drug. Anyone who has been on such treatment for a long period must therefore be weaned off the drug slowly. Sometimes this can be done with a combination of high potency vitamin B complex with vitamin C plus a herbal tranquillizer.

Pain-killing drugs

A common feature of most, though not all, nerve problems is the presence of pain. Pain is the most common symptom for which people seek help. It can reflect either physical or emotional discomfort. Physical pain is the result of tissue injury and arises from stimulation of specific pain nerves in all parts of the body. Psychogenic pains arise from chronic muscle tension or may simply originate in the person's imagination. They most frequently arise in the head, the abdomen or the low back.

Although management of the cause of the pain is the prime consideration, until this is diagnosed therapy to remove the pain itself is usually indicated. Sometimes simple rest of the painful part, application of hot or cold compresses or even a change in physical position is sufficient to relieve the pain. More often than not, however, a pain-killing drug (or analgesic) is sought, which usually removes the pain by depressing the peripheral sensory nerves.

Analgesics fall roughly into two types; those that relieve mild or moderate pain and those that are used to treat severe pain. The latter are called narcotic analgesics. There are many analgesics available but for the purposes of this book we shall examine just two of them, aspirin and paracetamol. Both are available on general sale since they fall into the mild category. The stronger analgesics are prescription-only and beyond the scope of this book.

Aspirin

This is the everyday name for the drug acetylsalicylic acid. World production runs into hundreds of thousands of tonnes per year. When you consider that a tablet usually contains only 300mg (or just less than one-third of 1g) and 1 tonne is 1 million grams, total consumption of aspirin as tablets runs into billions. In the USA alone, about 20 billion aspirin tablets are taken annually which works out at 100 per head of population. Annual intakes of all other western countries and Australasia are also close to this figure of 100 tablets per head of population.

Aspirin suppresses headache temporarily but the cause remains untreated, hence the danger of its continued use. In addition, the use of aspirin tends to neutralize vitamins in the body and often leads to digestive upsets. It also leaves a residue of chemical matter in the stomach which cannot be assimilated. This residue is carried by the bloodstream to the kidneys where it has an irritating effect upon the sensitive membranes lining the kidney tubules, and can cause permanent stomach disorder and kidney weakness. It is advisable to seek the cause of your headache, rather than benumb its effect with drugs. Headaches can arise from constipation, stomach upsets, sluggish liver, nervous tension, low blood sugar, high blood-pressure, anaemia, eye trouble, sinusitis, migraine and many other causes. Although we tend to use aspirin for headaches, it is also taken for all other types of pain produced by nerve problems.

Aspirin at ordinary recommended doses will not produce visible side-effects but one of these is important because it involves irritation of the gastric (stomach) lining. This in turn leads to dyspepsia, gastric lining erosion, ulceration, bleeding from the site and sometimes even vomiting of blood.

Slight blood loss occurs in about 70 per cent of those who take aspirin. Regular aspirin-taking can thus eventually lead to anaemia.

Asthmatics, amongst others, can exhibit high sensitivity to aspirin. The results can be skin rashes, water retention, rhinitis, and occasionally an asthmatic attack.

Mild symptoms of intoxication with aspirin can include dizziness, tinnitus (ringing in the ears), sweating, nausea, vomiting and mental confusion. More severe signs include fever and depression of the central nervous system leading to coma, heart circulation problems and respiratory failure. An adult toxic dose of aspirin drug is 25-30g, which can be fatal.

It has been known since 1936 that aspirin can interfere with vitamin C utilization. It increases the urinary excretion of the vitamin. Two aspirin tablets taken every six hours by healthy subjects double the loss of the vitamin in the urine over that twenty-four hours. Studies reported in the *Lancet* in 1973 concluded that between 200 and 300mg of vitamin C should be taken for every aspirin swallowed.

Vitamin C can confer other benefits in those taking aspirin apart from simple replacement of the lost vitamin. The efficacy of aspirin absorption is increased by giving vitamin C at the same time as the aspirin is taken. This in turn leads to earlier pain relief, slower excretion and longer duration of the drug. At the same time the gastric discomfort, blood loss and sedation induced by aspirin are reduced by vitamin C. A study reported in the *Lancet* in 1968 indicated that aspirin is more likely to cause gastric bleeding in those people who have low vitamin C body levels.

It would therefore appear to be a wise precaution to take supplementary vitamin C when aspirin therapy is undertaken. This is of particular importance when the drug is taken for prolonged periods in some nerve diseases and in inflammatory conditions like arthritis.

Paracetamol

Paracetamol is rapidly catching up with aspirin in its popular use as a readily-available analgesic. One reason is the lack of gastric bleeding with paracetamol but this is tempered by an increased chance of liver disease with the drug. This effect can be an insidious one, even on relatively low doses if they are taken over prolonged periods.

Visible side-effects of paracetamol are usually mild ones, like skin eruptions, although there have been reports of blood problems. An overdose of paracetamol causes death, usually through liver and kidney failure. Nevertheless, the drug is usually regarded as being safer than aspirin.

There have been reports in medical literature that the insidious side-effects of paracetamol can be reduced by increased intakes of vitamin E. This protective effect of the vitamin is probably mediated through increased production of substances in the liver that prevent paracetamol and its products from attacking liver cells. It could therefore be prudent to ensure that when taking paracetamol on a regular basis, natural vitamin E at the rate of 100 i.u. with each meal is also taken. Vitamin E is stored in the liver and the fatty tissues so its protective action is more prolonged.

Herbal Treatments for Nerve Complaints

Many herbal products are specific hypnotics, sedatives and analgesics, but unlike their drug counterparts they are perfectly safe when taken at the recommended dosage. In most commercially available herbal preparations for insomnia, these herbs are in combination since complementary actions are often a feature of herbal therapy. The following herbs for the nerves are all available in the UK for general sale. In some people a single herb such as Passiflora is often sufficient.

Cypripedium, also known as Lady's Slipper, Nerve Root and American Valerian, is particularly useful when combined with Humulus, also known as Hops, in treating insomnia due to depression. For anxiety states a combination with Avena (oats) or with Scutellaria (Skullcap) is particularly effective.

Passiflora or Passion Flower is an excellent hypnotic and sedative with specific indication in neuralgia. When combined with Valerian and Humulus, it is often used to treat insomnia. Valerian, of course, is one of the best herbal tranquillizers when used alone. Piscidia (or Jamaican Dogwood) acts as a sedative in treating neuralgia or nervous tension. Like Passiflora it has an enhanced effect when taken in combination with Humulus and Valerian.

Pulsatilla, also known as Prairie Anemone, is widely used in treating all types of nerve conditions but, unlike many other herbs, it possesses pain-killing or analgesic properties. On its own it is specific as a sedative and analgesic in painful conditions of the male and female reproductive systems. In combination with Passiflora, it can be used to treat headache and nervous excitability, so acting as a mild tranquillizer.

Migraine has many causes, including worry, stress and anxiety. Although simple analgesics like those mentioned above (both drug and herbal) can help relieve the pain of the condition, there is a herbal remedy that goes one step further, and prevents the migraine attack in the first place. Feverfew has been used for centuries to lower the temperature in feverish conditions but recently its specific properties have been utilized in migraine prevention. When taken on a regular basis, the dried leaf, or the fresh leaf if you have access to the plant, has this prophylactic action. It is believed to function through action of its constituents in the blood platelets (tiny white cells) by inhibiting the release of substances believed to trigger off the migraine attack.

Feverfew is a powerful herb and warnings have appeared recently in the medical press about the highly potent activity of its constituents. For this reason it is recommended that no more than two 25mg of dried herb leaf should be taken daily in preventing migraine. One small leaf, about 1 inch in diameter, will provide approximately 25mg dried powder. The herb is not recommended to be taken during pregnancy because it has not been studied sufficiently in this condition. It may also have abortifacient properties which can cause harm to the growing foetus.

These are only a few of the herbs known to provide relief in many nerve troubles. You can find out more about these and other herbal remedies from the many excellent books on herbal medicine that are now available.

5

Nerves and the Vitamin B Complex

The term 'nerves', although used frequently by lay people, has no meaning in medical terminology. It usually applies to the mild irritations, depressions, excitability and so on that represent vague symptoms and that are invariably treated with the libriums, valiums and other tranquillizers beloved by the medical profession. However, many of these nervous conditions will respond to members of the vitamin B complex. The reason for this is that the functions of these vitamins, and indeed of vitamin C, are intimately concerned with maintaining healthy nerves. It is possible, too, that the tranquillizing drugs are also upsetting our use of the B vitamins so we are in fact creating a vicious circle.

The three vitamins, thiamine (B_1), riboflavin (B_2) and nicotinamide (sometimes known as B_3) are all concerned in producing energy from carbohydrates (starches and sugars) in the diet. Carbohydrates represent the main, if not the only, source of energy for nerves. Hence any deficiency in these vitamins will reflect in abnormal nerve metabolism which leads to the condition we know as 'nerves'. Brain cells are nourished in the same way so perhaps it is not surprising that lack of these vitamins produces dementia, forgetfulness, and so on.

Vitamin B_6 is known as the anti-depression vitamin because lack of it induces mild depression. All nerves perform their function by secreting tiny amounts of specific chemical compounds at their nerve ends. The production of these substances is under the control of B_6 so in its absence they are not produced and the nerves cease to function correctly.

Vitamin B_{12} and folic acid are usually regarded as the anti-anaemia vitamins but they also serve other functions. For example, B_{12} is required to maintain a healthy myelin sheath; in the absence of the vitamin the nerves are not properly insulated and produce abnormal responses. Lack of these vitamins invariably causes nerve problems as well as anaemia.

Two other members of the B complex, pantothenic acid and biotin, exert their action on the nerves indirectly through the hormone-producing glands of the body. Lack of the vitamins induces stress which is the prime arbiter of many of the milder nervous complaints. Choline and inositol, which are present in lecithin, also contribute to the health of the fatty myelin sheath that surrounds nerves. Choline is the precursor of the active substance that is released in the brain, and it is now suspected that lack of choline is one of the causes of dementia in the elderly. Treatment with choline or lecithin often results in alleviation of the condition and even helps in cases of forgetfulness.

We can see, therefore, how important all of the B vitamins are in maintaining a healthy nervous system. This is the one common factor that links these vitamins as a complex. Let us therefore discuss in more detail how each of the B vitamins contributes to the upkeep of healthy nerves and brain. We shall also see the reasons why a mild deficiency of these vitamins can occur—a deficiency that can contribute to many of the nerve complaints we see today.

As we have seen, the first three members of the vitamin B complex, thiamine (vitamin B_1), riboflavin (vitamin B_2) and nicotinamide (also known as vitamin B_3, niacinamide, niacin, or nicotinic acid) are the energy vitamins, which means that they have an essential function in converting the foodstuffs we eat to the energy we need to sustain life. Nerves and the brain are only able to utilize glucose as an energy source. The energy vitamins are essential co-factors or co-enzymes in the burning of glucose to produce energy for the nerves.

Thiamine (Vitamin B_1)

Glucose is converted to energy via a compound known as pyruvic acid which is fed into the energy (or tricarboxylic acid) cycle. When thiamine is lacking, pyruvic acid builds up in the body and in the blood and these high levels produce profound changes. There is loss of appetite, easy fatigue, nausea, muscle weakness, and digestive upsets. There are also mental disturbances including a loss of mental alertness, with emotional disturbances such as depression, irritability, impairment of memory, and a reduction in the powers of concentration.

These symptoms have been observed in those suffering from a gross deficiency of thiamine leading to the disease beri-beri and they reflect the dependence of the nervous system on glucose as its main source of energy. However, even in milder states of deficiency (in volunteers deliberately deprived of the vitamin) the memory becomes faulty and the concentration poor. The individual becomes emotionally unstable, over-reacting to normal stresses and strains.

Eventually the nervous symptoms get worse, resulting in a tingling and burning in the toes and soles of the feet with the calves becoming extremely tender. The effects of thiamine deficiency on the brain and nervous system result in personality changes appearing long before other more obvious symptoms not connected with the nerves.

People whose intake of thiamine is inadequate may suffer from poor memory, lack of initiative, confused thinking, and frequently from depression and fear. The reason is that the brain cells depend upon blood sugar for their energy and blood sugar, as we have seen, cannot be transformed into energy without thiamine. Moreover, the accumulation of pyruvic and lactic acids which follows a poor supply of thiamine has a toxic effect upon brain cells. Tests carried out by American medical scientists put this matter beyond doubt. Professor E. V. McCollum, in *The Newer Knowledge of Nutrition*, states: 'Some of the nervous symptoms of thiamine deficiency in humans are numbness and tingling sensations, particularly affecting the fingers and usually associated with a gnawing pain which runs up the arms, especially at night.' This tingling sensation is of the 'pins and needles' type.

Studies on Children

The essential function of thiamine in nerve and brain function has been demonstrated by Dr R. F. Harvell of Columbia University in children between the ages of 9 and 19 years. The children, all on diets believed to be adequate in thiamine, were divided into two groups. One group was given 2mg supplementary thiamine daily; the others only received thiamine from their diet. After one year, those receiving the extra thiamine exhibited a large increase in mental achievements using the criteria of mental alertness, emotional stability, lack of depression and zest for life. No child in either group showed symptoms of thiamine deficiency before or after the trial.

How can mild deficiencies of thiamine arise? One of the most likely factors that affects all of us is an increasing intake of refined and processed foods that have been robbed of thiamine. This starvation began some ninety years ago when the refining of flour was introduced. The B-complex vitamins are in the husks of grain, and the refining process removes the husks and leaves a white flour, but a flour of reduced dietetic value.

The purpose of refining flour was to prevent it from going rancid. Wholemeal flour was a problem. Either it went rancid in store or when shipped overseas, weevils, rats and mice got into it. Then it was discovered that it was the wheatgerm oil in the husk that was responsible for the rancidity, and after much research machines were invented which separated the husk from the flour. The resultant product—a beautiful white flour—would not go rancid, no matter how long it was stored, and it was also less susceptible to infestation from pests. But people knew little about food values in those days and in their ignorance white flour became the basic universal food. Moreover, the white appearance of flour was attributed to its 'purity' and it was held to be much superior to ordinary wholemeal flour, which has a brownish colour. Thus science dealt the human race a mortal blow. The world began to 'live' on bread and flour products which were deficient in vitamin E (that also comes from the germ cell of grain) and some twelve of the B-complex vitamins. From that point onward the incidence of heart disease, nervous disorders, and a dozen other related diseases increased appallingly. It has been pointed out by Dr Haven Emerson, of Columbia

University, that since grains were first refined, diabetes has increased 1150 per cent, heart diseases 1200 per cent, and nervous disorders have increased to astronomical proportions.

Excessive consumption of refined carbohydrates can induce deficiency of thiamine because removal of the vitamin upsets the balance between carbohydrate and B_1 intakes. As a general rule, the more carbohydrate that is eaten, the more thiamine is needed. If more thiamine is not taken, the mild nervous upsets described above will appear. For various reasons the elderly and those who are pregnant or breast-feeding will need more because their condition demands it. Fever and surgery and other stressful conditions also cause increased requirements. Hence if all these individuals do not take extra thiamine, mild deficiency will result.

Alcohol may exert a deleterious effect upon the body levels of thiamine, so much so that in heavy drinkers there is a condition called alcoholic beri-beri where gross deficiency is induced by a combination of poor diet and alcohol. A feature of alcoholic beri-beri is an alcoholic neuropathy which can occur even in moderate drinkers, indicating that it does not require a gross deficiency of the vitamin for nerve symptoms to appear. Some authorities are so concerned with this effect of alcohol that they are studying the possibility of adding vitamin B_1 to wines and spirits.

Thiamine is unstable, particularly in the presence of alkalis such as in baking powders. Using them in baking can cause up to 50 per cent destruction of the vitamin. Soda, too, can be harmful when added to vegetables prior to boiling. Sulphur dioxide, used in preserving fruit and vegetables and in retaining the colour of fresh meat, will destroy virtually all of the vitamins.

Cooking methods will cause some destruction of thiamine

but most losses are by simple leaching into the cooking fluids because of the water solubility of the vitamin. These losses are easily recovered by using those fluids in gravy, sauces and the like.

Vitamin B_1 is widely distributed in foods but is particularly rich in wholegrains, pulses, nuts, green and root vegetables and dairy products (except butter). Organ meats like liver, kidney and heart are excellent sources, as are yeast and yeast extracts.

Riboflavin (Vitamin B_2)

This vitamin provides energy by acting as a co-enzyme in the oxidation of amino acids (from protein), of fatty acids (from fat) and of sugars (from starches). Riboflavin acts in body cell respiration to ensure efficient utilization of oxygen. Like thiamine, it is essential for the burning of sugars by nerves but the manifestations of deficiency on the nerves are not as clear-cut as with thiamine. Hence when riboflavin is lacking, trembling, dizziness, insomnia and a slow mental attitude have been noted.

Vitamin B_2 is a water-soluble vitamin which loses its potency when exposed to the light. It cannot be stored in the body. This vitamin is beneficial for sores or cracks at the corners of the mouth, burning and dryness (or watering) of the eyes, disorders of the cornea, burning sensation of the feet, trembling and 'twilight' blindness. It is also useful for cataract (in conjunction with vitamins C and E).

Riboflavin is likely to be deficient in the diet for the same reasons as those mentioned above for thiamine. However, light is the great destroyer of the vitamin, particularly in milk that has been exposed to sunlight. Heat is likely to destroy it only in the presence of alkali.

The most important sources of riboflavin are liver, milk and dairy products, eggs, and green vegetables. Grains, flours and cereals are not particularly good providers (unlike most of the other B vitamins) but they are often fortified with the vitamin. Yeast extract remains the best source because in it the vitamin is concentrated from the original yeast cells that provide it.

Nicotinamide (Vitamin B$_3$)

Nicotinamide is also known as niacinamide, nicotinic acid or niacin. It functions in the production of energy as an integral part of two co-enzymes called NAD (nicotinamide adenine dinucleotide) and NADP (nicotinamide adenine dinucleotide phosphate). These co-enzymes assist in the breakdown and utilization of carbohydrates, fats and protein. They thus occupy a central role in the production of energy in the nerve and other tissues and in maintaining their health. The vitamin is therefore essential for the proper utilization of the brain and nervous system in addition to maintaining a healthy skin, tongue and digestive organs.

Gross deficiency of nicotinamide (or of nicotinic acid, which is how it occurs in foods) leads to the disease pellagra, characterized by the three D's, dermatitis, diarrhoea and dementia, leading eventually to the fourth, death. In the early stages of deficiency there is muscular weakness, general fatigue, loss of appetite, indigestion and minor skin complaints. Nerve problems include insomnia, irritability, stress and depression. Upsets in the digestive tract are characterized by nausea, vomiting and an inflamed mouth and gastro-intestinal system.

In a mild deficiency of nicotinic acid the tongue is usually a bright red at the tip, but further back it is coated. A furred tongue and bad breath often indicate a lack of nicotinic acid. When canker sores and small ulcers form on the cheeks or under the tongue there is every likelihood that the niacin intake is inadequate. A mild lack of nicotinic acid causes digestive disturbances, because the secretion of hydrochloric acid in the stomach diminishes and stomach trouble follows. As this stomach acid is required to promote the assimilation of vitamin C, protein, iron and calcium, anaemia and nerve disorders can result. With the digestive system disorganized, food is not properly absorbed, causing flatulence, constipation or diarrhoea. Gradually the entire intestinal tract becomes inflamed, noticeably in the region of the rectum and anus. Unless this condition is rectified, it may lead to colitis. A deficiency of nicotinic acid can also cause dizziness, insomnia, irritability, nausea, vomiting and recurring headaches. In more severe deficiencies there is a sensation of strain, tension, and deep depression. For the last two centuries, the disease known as pellagra, from pelle agra, meaning rough skin, has occurred fairly constantly in districts where maize is the staple item of food. It is now known that maize is deficient in tryptophan, an essential amino acid which is a precursor of nicotinic acid. The conversion of tryptophan to nicotinic acid is considered to occur in the tissues, not as a result of the action of intestinal micro-organisms.

Nicotinic acid is present in almost all the tissues, chiefly as a co-enzyme and more is contained in the liver than in any other organ. Chronic alcoholics and those with serious liver ailments may have difficulty in storing niacin because of this fact. Nicotinic acid is resistant to oxygen in the air and also to the heat of cooking but, like riboflavin, it is easily leached away in the water used for cooking.

Sources of nicotinic acid

The foods richest in nicotinic acid are liver, meat, fish, yeast and wheatgerm. Other foods containing nicotinic acid are eggs, nuts, and wheat bran. There is practically none in white flour. Nicotinic acid deficiency can be produced by the use of sulphonamide drugs, and by antibiotics such as penicillin. Alcohol is also notorious for inducing nicotinic acid deficiency. Like the other B-complex vitamins, food refining and processing is a major factor in removing the vitamin from the foods as grown.

Schizophrenia

The mental symptoms associated with nicotinic acid deficiency are similar to those seen in schizophrenia and include tension, depression, personality problems and mental fatigue. Such observations have stimulated many doctors, including the pioneers Drs H. Osmond, A. Hoffer, A. Cott and D. Hawkins, to treat schizophrenia with high doses of nicotinic acid and other vitamins, an approach now known as megavitamin therapy or orthomolecular medicine. High doses mean daily intakes of nicotinic acid or nicotinamide—up to 5g, which is some 250 times the amount in an average diet.

No one should attempt self-treatment with these massive doses of vitamins since each person requires individual intakes tailored to them and dependent on other treatment. This particularly applies to treating schizophrenia in children. The advice of a doctor sympathetic to orthomolecular medicine must be sought since only he or she can institute complete therapy.

Alcoholics often exhibit mental symptoms similar to those in schizophrenics and are treated with megadose vitamins in a similar fashion. Some success has been reported by Dr R. F. Smith of Michigan. There are also claims that moderately high intakes of nicotinamide or nicotinic acid can help stop tobacco addicts from smoking. Despite the similarity in names, nicotinic acid is not related in any way to nicotine.

Pyridoxine (Vitamin B_6)

Pyridoxine is known as the 'anti-depression' vitamin because of its role in the production of brain substances, lack of which may induce a state of mild depression. The vitamin has many functions but here we are concerned with its co-enzymic property in the conversion of amino acids derived from the food into brain constituents that play their part in controlling both brain and nerve functions.

One of these amino acids is called L-tryptophan and under the control of pyridoxine it is converted into the other B-complex vitamin, nicotinic acid. We have seen how important this vitamin is in maintaining healthy nerves so pyridoxine is indirectly involved too. The other product from L-tryptophan which is synthesized under the influence of pyridoxine is serotonin. This substance is produced constantly in the brain and at nerve endings. When production is deficient, the results are a form of depression and sleep disturbances. The control of mood is dependent on adequate brain concentrations of serotonin. Hence anything that interferes with these will manifest itself as a mental or nervous problem. Pyridoxine is therefore at the hub of nervous control.

There are two conditions where increased requirements for pyridoxine are needed. If these are not supplied the result is an upset in L-tryptophan metabolism with a lowering of serotonin brain levels. The first occurs in many women who are taking the contraceptive pill. The second is in those women who suffer from premenstrual tension, whether or not they are taking the contraceptive pill.

Clinical trials carried out at St Mary's Hospital in London demonstrated that out of thirty-nine women with depression who were taking the Pill, nineteen had an absolute deficiency of pyridoxine. Administration of up to 40mg of the vitamin daily to these women removed the depressive state from which they suffered. It is believed that the synthetic oestrogen component of the Pill induced in its taker an increased requirement for the vitamin. In other words, the deficiency was artificially produced because the Pill was increasing requirements of pyridoxine over and above those available even from a good diet.

Premenstrual syndrome describes many symptoms that are suffered by some women ten days or so before they start to menstruate. Those symptoms that affect the mental and nervous systems fall into a sub-group complaint called premenstrual tension. This is characterized by nervous tension, mood swings, anxiety, irritability, headache, depression, confusion and insomnia, all complaints of the nervous system.

Studies at St Thomas's Hospital in London have indicated that many of these symptoms are relieved by simple supplementation with pyridoxine. Two regimes appear to be equally effective. In the first, 25 or 50mg of the vitamin is taken daily; in the second, 100mg of the vitamin is taken from day 10 of one menstrual cycle to day 3 of the next. A beneficial response was noted in 63 per cent of those undergoing the trial. Relief of premenstrual headache was enjoyed by over 80 per cent of those afflicted.

L-glutamic acid is another amino acid that is converted into an essential brain substance under the influence of pyridoxine. This substance is known as gamma-butyric acid (GABA) and it is a natural calming agent produced by the central nervous system. When it is lacking in the brain, convulsions can take place, so here again vitamin B_6 can be seen to be playing a part in nervous control. Some infants are particularly prone to vitamin B_6 deficiency, either because of a deficient intake in their milk or because they suffer a genetic defect where they cannot utilize the vitamin. In the former case, low level supplementation is sufficient; in the latter, more rare condition, relatively high levels of pyridoxine must be given under medical supervision.

The vitamin is widely distributed in foods but is particularly rich in liver, kidney, pork, veal, fish, bananas, avocados, prunes, raisins, walnuts and wholegrain cereals. It is stable to most cooking methods and most losses are due to leaching into cooking fluids from which it can be recovered. It does have a low stability in heated milk, however, but modern methods of dried milk production have been developed to lessen this loss. Low levels may be produced in the body by reaction with many medicinal drugs.

Pantothenic Acid

This is also known as vitamin B_5 and has been referred to as the anti-stress vitamin. The name reflects its importance in the adrenal gland where it functions in the production of anti-stress corticosteroid hormones from cholesterol. It does, however, perform many body functions as a co-enzyme in energy production; for fat and cholesterol metabolism; for antibody formation in resisting infection and in ensuring a healthy nervous system.

It is significant that the only deficiency symptom of lack of pantothenic acid in man is the 'burning feet' syndrome which would appear to be nervous in origin. The earliest symptoms are aching, burning or throbbing in the feet. These discomforts become more intense and develop into sharp, stabbing, shooting pains that may spread as far as the knee.

Studies on human volunteers deliberately deprived of the vitamin have indicated deficiency symptoms that include loss of appetite, indigestion, respiratory infections and reduced hormone production. Nerve complaints included abdominal pain, neuritis, cramps in the limbs, insomnia, fatigue and depression. Nervous disease and psychosis are well documented in alcoholics who lack the vitamin because of poor diet combined with the ill-effects of alcohol on pantothenic acid absorption and assimilation.

The name pantothenic acid is derived from the Greek word 'panthos' meaning everywhere and it was coined by its discoverer, Dr R. J. Williams of the University of Texas, to reflect its universal distribution in foods. Nevertheless, food processing and refining techniques cause irrecoverable losses of the vitamin and dry-processing of foods in particular is highly destructive. Cooking methods lead to losses by leaching but these can be recovered with a little thought. Deep-frozen foods can lose substantial amounts of pantothenic acid in storage but the reasons for this are not clear.

Substantial supplies of the vitamin are provided by the bacteria that inhabit the lower part of the bowel, so any factor that destroys these micro-organisms, such as antibiotic treatment, can cut off a useful source. Replenishment of these bacteria with live yogurt or freeze-dried in capsules can ensure that their pantothenic acid and other vitamin-producing capacity is restored.

Biotin

This is regarded as another anti-stress B vitamin but the effects of its deficiency on the nervous system are not as well reported as those of pantothenic acid. As it is required for energy production from carbohydrates, fats and protein it plays a part in providing energy for nerve cells. Lack of the vitamin is believed to induce stress in the individual, probably because like pantothenic acid it is concerned in the production of anti-stress hormones by the adrenal glands.

Biotin accompanies the rest of the B-vitamin complex in such varied foods as yeast, liver, eggs, fish, nuts, and wholegrains. Cooking methods tend to cause loss by leaching but destruction of the vitamin can occur during the drying of milks. Food processing and refining will also lead to losses from foods as they occur in nature.

Food sources may be less important than the quantities of biotin synthesized by the intestinal bacteria. Losses are therefore likely to occur when these bacteria are destroyed by antibiotics and the like. Raw egg white contains a protein, avidin, that combines with and immobilizes biotin, but such a reaction is unlikely to lead to a deficiency for most people, except for food faddists who have been known to exist solely on raw egg white.

Folic Acid

This B vitamin is known as an anti-anaemia vitamin since lack of it produces a typical macrocytic anaemia. This is characterized by abnormally large red blood cells. Studies also indicate that folic acid plays an important part in brain function.

One such study was reported from Massachusetts General Hospital in the 1975 *New England Journal of Medicine*. Some mentally retarded or disturbed patients responded favourably to folic acid treatment. Schizophrenics also received some benefits from the vitamin, losing some of their psychotic symptoms after high doses. Folic acid, like pyridoxine, is needed for the production of brain and nerve substances and this property explains its necessity for a healthy nervous system.

Confirmation came from Northwick Park Hospital, Harrow, in the UK, that schizophrenia and other mental conditions may respond to folic acid alone but doses were in the range 5mg to 20mg daily. These intakes are from ten to forty times what one could obtain from a really good diet.

Folic acid is also needed for proper development of the nervous system in the growing foetus. Recent studies suggest that low intakes of the vitamin during pregnancy increase the chances of the baby being born with spina bifida. In this condition part of the spinal cord is exposed through a gap in the backbone because the neural tube (which gives rise to the spinal cord) has not closed. Symptoms include nerve paralysis of the legs and mental retardation. A large-scale trial is at present being undertaken in the UK to determine if folic acid is the only factor in preventing spina bifida.

Nutritional folic acid deficiency is usually the result of poor diet combined with destructive cooking methods. The vitamin is also adversely affected by many medicinal drugs and by the ingredients of the contraceptive pill. Little wonder, then, that many people are on the borderline of deficiency.

Though folic acid is found in many foods, it can occur in a multiple of forms, not all of which can be utilized as a vitamin. The richest sources of active vitamin are provided by liver, oysters and yeast extracts but green large-leaf vegetables also contain significant amounts. Since up to 45 per cent of the vitamin can be lost from fruit and vegetables during cooking, the rule is to eat them raw when possible.

Vitamin B_{12}

Also known as cyanocobalamin and hydroxocobalamin, this too is an anti-anaemia vitamin. Lack of it causes a macrocytic anaemia called pernicious anaemia. It is similar in many respects to that found in folic acid deficiency. This is not surprising in view of the fact that the two vitamins work together in the production of red blood cells.

The essential difference between the two deficiencies lies in the effect on the central nervous system. When vitamin B_{12} is lacking there is an insidious and dangerous degeneration of the nerve fibres in the spinal cord and elsewhere. The lesion is essentially due to demyelination of these fibres. At the same time the brain is affected by the vitamin lack since psychosis with mental deterioration has also been reported.

Since the macrocytic anaemia can appear before nerve degeneration, lack of vitamin B_{12} can sometimes be regarded just as folic acid deficiency. Those with high intakes of folic acid, such as vegetarians, can therefore have their B_{12} deficiency masked by this folic acid since the anaemia will not appear but nerve degeneration will continue. This makes it imperative that any macrocytic anaemia is diagnosed and treated professionally.

Such tiny amounts of vitamin B_{12} are needed daily that dietary deficiency is unlikely. At the same time, since the vitamin is confined to foodstuffs of animal origin, some vegetarians, and vegans in particular, may be prone to dietary deficiency. In these cases oral supplementation becomes essential. Usually, however, lack of vitamin B_{12} is a result of an inability to absorb even the tiny amounts found in the diet. When malabsorption is the problem, medical treatment has to be sought because the vitamin must then be given by intramuscular injection.

6

Nerves and Other Nutrients

We have seen that an adequate daily intake of the vitamin B complex is essential for maintaining a healthy nervous system, but other vitamins and minerals also play their part in keeping the central nervous system and the brain healthy. Deficiency of these other nutrients can also induce changes in the nervous system leading to specific complaints that can only be cured by replacing the vitamin or mineral that is lacking. Stress is one of most common factors in causing nerve problems and, as we shall see, this stress can bring about a greater need for certain vitamins and minerals in the sufferer.

Vitamin C (Ascorbic Acid)

Early indications that stress conditions induce extra requirements for vitamin C came from experimental studies on animals. Typical stress factors included loud noises, flashing lights, extreme heat or cold, electric shock, irradiation (including x-rays), drugs, chemicals, infections with bacteria or viruses, surgical operation, accidents, fasting, immobility, excessive exercise, and inhalation or feeding of toxic substances—in fact, all the conditions that most people will meet at some times in their lives. What emerged was that inadequate intakes of vitamin C reduced the animals' ability to withstand stress, but giving large doses of the vitamin protected them.

Those animals who could not withstand stress and died were found to have adrenal glands that were literally exhausted. The anti-stress hormones produced normally by these glands were no longer available to help the animals withstand stress and this is why they succumbed. A study in old people who were diagnosed as having 'exhausted' adrenal glands indicated that a daily intake of 500mg of vitamin C stimulated production of the adrenal anti-stress hormones.

As we have already seen, links between vitamin C and stress had been made much earlier than this. Dr James Lind in 1753, reported that scurvy (due to lack of vitamin C) was more liable to break out in ships where the crews were exposed to the stresses induced by cold and damp working conditions; rough seas with the threat of sinking; fatigue and debilitation by other diseases. In other words, these stressful conditions induced a greater requirement for vitamin C that was not met by the poor diets of these sailors.

Two hundred years later, these observations were also made on other explorers, the first astronauts. Although the dietary requirements of these people had been worked out carefully, their vitamin and mineral contents were based on those needed for normal living conditions. When they returned to earth, these astronauts were found to have low blood and body levels of most of the vitamins, including vitamin C. No one had allowed for the severe mental stress that these pioneers were undergoing. This lack of forethought was reflected in their body vitamin status. Needless to say, later astronauts were fed extra vitamins and minerals and their body status of these micro-nutrients remained high.

Not many of us will experience the strains and stresses of space flight, but similar factors are a feature of everyday life. All can deplete us of vitamin C and the members of the B-complex. An improved diet, with supplementation of these vitamins if necessary, will provide the extra requirements to help us cope.

Vitamin E (d-alpha tocopherol)

The nervous system can be adversely affected when vitamin E is lacking, and like so many observations, this was made on poultry deprived of the vitamin. A particular disease, known as encephalomalacia or softening of the brain, develops due to a restricted blood supply to that organ. This complaint, known as Crazy Chick Disease, is characterized by an inability of the bird to hold its head upright because the nerves supplying the muscles have degenerated. Mental confusion in the elderly person can sometimes be associated with low vitamin E levels in a similar manner. In both cases the disease can be relieved with vitamin E therapy.

There are three independent lines of evidence indicating that vitamin E is important for normal functioning of the nervous system in man, according to a leading article in the *Lancet* (1983). The first comes from study of a rare hereditary disease called abetalipoproteinaemia. Those suffering from the complaint are unable to carry vitamin E in the blood because they lack a specific protein-carrier called apoprotein B. At the same time there is a reduced efficacy in absorption of vitamin E, with the result that blood vitamin E levels are so low as to be undetectable.

Various things happened in these people but two particular conditions arose. There was a progressive degeneration of the nervous system and of the retina of the eye. The conditions were reversed only by massive oral doses or intramuscular injections of vitamin E. Nerve degeneration was halted or prevented and the retina regained normality. Constant therapy with vitamin E was necessary to allow these people to live normal lives.

The second approach was to study those individuals who cannot absorb vitamin E by the normal channels. These are people with chronic liver disease, cystic fibrosis, and those who have had surgical removal of parts of the intestine. The common factor was an inability to produce sufficient bile salts for vitamin E absorption and the common symptom was incoordination of muscular movement because of nerve degeneration. This led to lack of reflexes, impaired sense of position, muscle weakness and paralysis of the eye muscles. As the complaints are due to malabsorption of vitamin E, the only therapy is with injections of the vitamin. Treatment with water-solubilized vitamin E given orally is now showing promise.

The third line of study comes from vitamin E deficiency in rats and monkeys. These animals develop exactly the same nerve and muscle symptoms as those observed in human beings who cannot absorb vitamin E. What happens in all cases is a degeneration of the nerve axons, which are those areas at the ends of nerves that allow nerve impulses to be transmitted between nerve cells and between nerves and muscles.

Proof that vitamin E can help in treating nerve degeneration as described above has been presented by Dr J. H. Sung and colleagues in the *Journal of Neuropathological and Experimental Neurology* (1980). They found a fall in the incidence of nerve degeneration in those suffering from cystic fibrosis who died between 1979 and 1980 compared to those who died in the years 1952-1969, coincided with the introduction of vitamin E treatment for the disease in the mid 1960's. It is likely that vitamin E functions by maintaining a healthy myelin sheath that is essential for a normal nervous system.

Stress can also cause increased requirements for vitamin E. Studies reported by the National Aeronautics and Space Administration (NASA) indicated that the early astronauts lost up to 20 per cent of their red blood cells during space flights. Vitamin E is known to function in maintaining healthy red blood cells—when the vitamin is lacking, they tend to burst easily. Once a red cell has burst, its haemoglobin is lost to the blood plasma and it can no longer carry oxygen. Hence excessive breakdown of the red blood cells can cause a haemolytic anaemia which can be serious.

Later astronauts were given supplementary vitamin E in their pre-packed meals and the problem of red blood cell loss due to haemolysis disappeared. These experiences must make all of us aware of the danger of eating too many devitalized foods that have been deprived of their vitamin E. The vitamin is also lost to varying degrees during the storage of deep-frozen foods.

Iodine

The B-complex vitamins have a particularly important duty to perform. They help keep the ductless glands of the body's endocrine system in good condition, particularly that most important gland, the thyroid. A healthy thyroid gland depends primarily upon two main ingredients, a tiny amount of iodine each day (obtainable from sea food or kelp tablets) and adequate B-complex vitamins. Three or four B-complex tablets daily will suffice if your diet lacks this vitamin, which it probably does.

The Thyroid Gland

Some women are subject to a nervous condition that arises from the thyroid gland and which necessitates a medical examination. The thyroid gland has a powerful influence upon the texture and colour of the skin and hair, whether you are to be stout or thin, active or sluggish, languid or forceful. This gland consists of two lobes, one on each side of the windpipe at the base of the neck. The gland secretes and discharges into the blood stream a potent hormone called 'thyroxin', of which iodine is an essential constituent. If there is a deficiency of iodine in the diet, the normal functioning of the thyroid gland is upset and this can have disastrous results on the health.

The work of this gland is of the utmost importance because it regulates the metabolism of the body; that is, the continual chemical change that is going on whereby food is converted into energy, and various complex chemical substances are broken down into simple ones. The thyroid gland regulates the energy discharge of the body, maintains its normal temperature of 98.6°F, and exerts an important influence upon all the other glands in the endocrine system. According to Dr D. T. Quigley, once every seventeen minutes the entire volume of blood in the body passes through the thyroid gland and becomes charged with its secretions. This authority states that the thyroid gland evidently also acts as a trap for filtering out toxic matter, including low-grade micro-organisms in the bloodstream, because the iodine acts as an anti-toxin.

A partial lack of iodine causes goitre, which is an enlargement of the thyroid gland. This enlargement is an attempt on the part of the gland to compensate for the lack of iodine and use the inadequate supply more efficiently. The gland overworks in trying to secrete more thyroxin than it has the ingredient (iodine) to do it with. The result is that it enlarges and causes pressure and fullness of the neck, which is a danger signal. Goitre occurs frequently during adolescence when the body's need for iodine is greatest, and is much more prevalent among girls than boys.

Puberty, pregnancy, childbirth, and the menopause are conditions that require more thyroxin than usual, and so the thyroid gland is often slightly enlarged at these times. After the emergency is over, the gland may decrease in size, or continue to grow, especially if not enough iodine is present. In cases of simple goitre the gland may still manage to manufacture enough thyroxin to prevent visible signs, such as a swollen throat and bulging eyes, but there may be difficulty in swallowing, hoarseness, coughing and laboured breathing.

The Need for Iodine

When an iodine deficiency causes the thyroid gland to produce too little thyroxin (which is about 64 per cent iodine), the person becomes lazy, has no endurance, and puts on weight easily. Decreased energy causes the heart to slow down, and the person has poor circulation, with cold hands and feet, lifeless hair that lacks lustre and falls out easily, and thin fingernails that split and break readily. The memory is often faulty, owing to bad circulation of blood to the brain, and there are frequent headaches. The bone marrow may also fail to produce enough red cells. The result is anaemia, leading to even greater fatigue.

Recent surveys in America indicate that 40 per cent of the women in many communities are suffering from abnormally low production of thyroxin, leading to some or all of the above symptoms. There is no reason to believe that conditions are any better in Australia and New Zealand or in Europe.

The usual treatment for this condition, which is commonly called 'thyroid deficiency', is to administer thyroid tablets containing thyroxin. The tablets contain the thyroxin taken from the thyroid glands of sheep. When these tablets are taken for any length of time, the thyroid gland becomes unable to carry out its normal function. In effect, it is enfeebled, like an arm that has been kept in a sling. Hence the use of thyroid tablets is not recommended except in cases where the gland has been surgically removed. Thyroxin tablets, under medical direction, are then essential.

There is another form of goitre called 'exopthalmic' in which too much thyroxin is produced by the thyroid gland. In such cases all the bodily processes are speeded up. The heart beats too rapidly; the patient loses weight under the strain, becomes extremely nervous and suffers greatly from the heat. The eyes protrude from their sockets. Moreover, food is forced so rapidly through the digestive tract that it is not absorbed properly, and the person becomes ill-nourished despite all she eats. Some people find it impossible to relax because their nerves are in a state of continual tension, and unless they receive careful treatment their complaint can prove fatal.

Quite apart from iodine, vitamins A, B-complex, and C are important for the proper functioning of the thyroid gland.

A deficiency of these vitamins can cause a serious decrease in the output of thyroxin. The body requires approximately 0.1mg of iodine daily to remain healthy. The richest source of organic iodine is kelp, a type of seaweed obtained from the Pacific Ocean. Tincture of iodine, prepared as an antiseptic for external use, is a poison and should never be used internally. Goitre occurs naturally in certain localities where there is not enough iodine in the soil and the drinking water. These areas are known as 'goitre belts'. The prevention of goitre is a simple matter: three kelp tablets a day contain sufficient iodine to give immunity.

The remedy for goitre, whether it be caused by thyroid deficiency or an over-active thyroid, is a more difficult matter. In such cases, the thyroid gland must be made to function normally again. Foods rich in organic iron help to combat the anaemic condition associated with a sluggish thyroid. These are: apricots, prunes, dates, dried fruits, molasses, liver, egg yolk, and wheatgerm. The diet must also include such vital foods as fresh fruit and vegetables, cheese and milk, and you should eliminate the demineralized and refined foods that contain little or no nutritive value. Supplementary vitamins should comprise vitamin A tablets, vitamin C (250mg) tablets, vitamin B_1 (10mg) tablets, vitamin B-complex tablets, kelp, and calcium (white) tablets. One of each of the vitamin tablets should be taken three times daily before meals, with double dosages of the kelp and calcium tablets.

Calcium

We have seen how important vitamin B_1 and the other B-complex vitamins are in the treatment of nervous disorders, but that's not the whole story from a nutritional point of view. The diet must also be rich in calcium foods. Calcium is needed by every cell of the body. One writer calls calcium 'the prime instigator of vital activity'. Calcium is vital to the nerves because tiny particles of calcium called ions, which are atoms or groups of atoms, help in the transmission of nervous impulses. People who lack calcium feel tense and irritable. Children who are growing rapidly and whose bones require much calcium are often nervous and fretful for this reason. Adults are apt to be highly strung, bad tempered, and uneasy. They make mistakes in their work and quickly become fatigued. A lack of calcium can prevent a person from sleeping soundly, or he may awake during the night and find it difficult to sleep again. A few calcium tablets taken before retiring will often ensure a good night's sleep. Calcium helps to relax nerves and muscles and is always indicated in cramps and convulsions.

According to Professor Sir Stanton Hicks, an eminent Australian nutritional scientist, the Australian diet is likely to be deficient in calcium. When tissues lack calcium, this precious mineral is withdrawn from the teeth and bones. Soft, brittle bones are not just the natural result of old age—they suggest a lack of calcium in the diet. The blood cannot clot without calcium, so a slight scratch could prove fatal. Calcium is also needed to regulate the rhythmic beat of the heart.

Calcium requires an acid medium before the body can utilize it. This means that the gastric juice must contain an adequate amount of hydrochloric acid, or the calcium will remain insoluble and be lost to the body. Too much fat in the diet prevents the proper assimilation of calcium and too much phosphorus in the diet causes a less efficient utilization of calcium by the body.

Calcium Enemies

Cane sugar has a strong affinity for calcium and by uniting with it, prevents the body from making use of its calcium. Moreover sugar, which is acid, attacks the tooth enamel and causes dental decay. It also leads to arthritis and kindred ailments. Foods that contain oxalic acid, such as spinach and rhubarb, should be eaten sparingly, owing to this acid's destructive action upon calcium. Chocolate and cocoa also have an oxalic acid content.

Is there any danger of getting too much calcium? With all the talk nowadays about calcification, calcium deposits in arteries, and calcium in kidney stones, some may think that eating too much calcium could result in these misfortunes. The fact is that the body is excreting calcium all the time, whether there happens to be a calcium surplus or not. Any excess calcium is excreted, unless there is some disordered condition of the body that causes deposits of unassimilable calcium. The parathyroid glands (located in the neck) are responsible for the body's calcium management. If these glands are not functioning properly, calcium difficulties are indicated, but obviously the way to remedy such glandular disorder is not by eating more or less calcium, but with hormone therapy.

Vitamin D and Calcium

Calcium is largely retained in the body by being combined with phosphorus, and phosphorus and calcium cannot be absorbed efficiently without vitamin D. If the body is deficient in vitamin D, phosphorus cannot be utilized and part of the body's calcium, having no phosphorus to combine with, cannot be retained and so is excreted from the body.

In Australia, vitamin D is available for the greater part of the year to all who can take a walk in the sunshine. The ultra-violet rays in sunlight cause the oil glands of the skin to secrete a provitamin which is converted into vitamin D and absorbed into the body through the skin. People who cannot go out in the sunshine three or four times a week can obtain their vitamin D from vitamin A and D capsules, or from brown calcium tablets, which contain vitamin D.

Calcium and the Nerves

We have already seen that calcium plays a part in nerve impulse transmission by exchanging across the membrane of the nerve cell with magnesium. Lack of calcium can upset this balance and produce a condition called Tetany (not to be confused with Tetanus or lockjaw which is due to an infection). This is characterized by spasm and twitching of the muscles, particularly those of the face, hands and feet. The underlying problem is associated with the nervous system. Tetany is caused by a reduction in the blood calcium level which in turn can be due to underactive parathyroid glands or to rickets due to calcium and/or vitamin D deficiency.

Our Calcium Needs

The National Research Council of the USA considers that every child and every adult needs a minimum of 1g of calcium daily: 1g is equal to 1000mg. Pregnant women need 1500mg daily and growing children almost as much. The best natural sources of calcium are whole milk, dried skim-milk, and unprocessed cheese. Other good sources are chard, cabbage, cauliflower, beans, dates, broccoli, prunes, buttermilk, molasses, sardines, turnip tops (cooked), wheatgerm, egg yolk, dried figs, and lettuce.

Food refining and processing techniques cause serious losses of calcium from wholegrain cereals and in particular from wholewheat. White flour contains some 55 per cent less calcium than wholemeal flour. Although white flour is fortified with calcium by law in some countries, the mineral is usually added as chalk which may not be as well utilized as the calcium that has been removed from the original wholewheat flour.

Magnesium

Magnesium has been termed the best natural tranquillizer. This reputation is based on our knowledge of how magnesium combines with calcium in the transmission of nerve impulses. The important factor is the ratio of these minerals in the nerve cells. If this ratio is upset, nervous complications can arise. We have already seen how a low calcium level can lead to tetany.

When animals are fed on diets deficient in magnesium, they become extremely nervous and respond in an exaggerated manner to external stimuli such as noise and pain. These hypersensitivity reactions disappear when magnesium is given. When the mineral is deficient in man, the results are upsets in neuromuscular functions. The symptoms are high excitability, tremor and convulsions but there are also behavioural disturbances such as depression. Such conditions will often respond to increased magnesium intakes from the diet or by supplementation.

Like calcium, magnesium is readily removed from foods by refining and processing techniques. The mineral is widely distributed in foodstuffs but the less refined these are the more magnesium is available. Both minerals can conveniently be taken as dolomite, which supplies calcium and magnesium in the same ratio as that found in foods and regarded as the ideal. Calcium and magnesium are also present in such supplements as amino acid chelated minerals and also as gluconates. Both these forms are superior to conventional mineral salts in terms of their absorption by the body.

Zinc

When zinc is deficient in man, there is an important impact on mental function. Children who lack zinc are mentally lethargic, have poor concentration and are sullen, depressed, miserable, irritable, and tearful. They never smile or laugh, are difficult to soothe and refuse to be calmed by affection. When they are supplemented with zinc, the first sign of recovery is smiling, followed by other signs of normality.

One study carried out in the UK screened 112 patients admitted to hospital for psychiatric treatment for zinc and magnesium levels in the blood. All were low compared to controls. Sir MacFarlane Burnet, a leading doctor, has suggested in the *Lancet* (1981) that certain types of dementia may be associated with low levels of body zinc. He believes that administration of supplemental zinc could prevent or delay the development of dementia in those known to be at risk.

A paper by Dr J. Hart in the *Journal of Orthomolecular Psychiatry* reports that infants waking one or more times at night between midnight and 7 am improved their sleep pattern when given 12mg elemental zinc plus 1mg of manganese. After one week of this therapy on twenty-six infants, 76 per cent were sleeping through the night. At the same time, these infants demonstrated a reduction in irritability, diarrhoea and skin rashes, and their appetites improved. Dosage for infants should be 1mg of zinc for each kilogram of body weight.

Adults with any mental disturbance or behavioural or sleep disturbances could often profitably try zinc therapy. According to WHO reports, people are almost as likely to be deficient in zinc as they are in iron. As it is also readily removed by any processing or refining of foods, intakes may be low and these in turn could lead to many of the nervous and mental problems seen today.

The Importance of Lecithin

Lecithin, an essential food factor found in certain fatty foods, is essential to nerve health. No cell or body organ can function without lecithin, yet modern processing methods remove it from foods (edible oils). Lecithin is important to the nerve cells because it is a nerve food. The myelin sheath which surrounds each nerve is composed of a white, fatty substance rich in lecithin. This sheath not only protects and insulates the nerves, but also nourishes them. A high proportion of lecithin is needed to feed the brain, otherwise brain fag, nervous exhaustion and sleeplessness may follow. The richest sources of lecithin are vegetable and cereal oils, such as safflower seed oil, wheatgerm oil, sunflower seed oil, peanut oil, and soya bean oil, and capsules containing these oils are available.

According to a comprehensive report from the Food and Drug Administration of the USA (1981), lecithin may be useful in treating senile dementia and Alzheimer's disease in the aged. These complaints appear to be associated with degeneration of the brain leading to forgetfulness, absent-mindedness and loss of intellectual abilities. One factor in the development of dementia is a reduced capacity to produce the nerve substance (neurotransmitter) acetylcholine from its precursor, choline.

Lecithin is a rich source of choline and this is the reason why it can help some sufferers of these diseases to regain their full mental faculties. In some cases choline itself brought relief, but lecithin was preferred as the source of choline because it was less toxic at the high doses required. Lecithin also appeared to be better absorbed than pure choline.

7

Some Practical Examples

Nutrition and the Personality
A series of experiments lasting for six months was carried out at the University of Minnesota, USA. These experiments produced startling evidence of the havoc that nutritional deficiencies create on the human mind and personality. Details of the experiments are given in an article by J. R. Coggins in the *Rosicrucian Digest*. The article states that thirty-six male volunteers were put on a special restricted diet. The men were carefully selected for the rigorous test of prolonged hunger, due to an inadequate diet that also lacked vitamins and minerals.

Apathy was the first sign of mental deterioration; next came deep depression, until gradually more insidious factors began to reveal themselves; namely boredom, inability to concentrate, and loss of self-confidence. Eventually, all these characteristics became exaggerated into what was called semi-starvation neurosis. Sometimes, apathy was succeeded by frustrations and strong irritations, which, in the final stages of the experiment, revealed disturbances of mental balance. There was a total lack of sense of humour among the volunteers. Mistrust and resentment towards the research scientists conducting the experiment was the next sign. The men grew suspicious of each other. Self-doubt increased, and finally came feelings of persecution and a strong sense of martyrdom.

The diaries kept by the volunteers revealed mental confusion and even morbid, undefinable fear. One of the men became obsessed with the idea that there were stairs he must climb, when there actually were not any. In his weakening condition, this obsession became a form of self-torture. The research doctors dared not carry the experiment any further, as the human stresses had become almost unbearable. But much had been learned that would more than compensate for the sacrifices made by the volunteers.

It was proved that deficiency of vitamin B_1 alone produces listlessness and a mild form of mental and emotional disorganization. Vitamin B_1 is essential to the integration of the personality, and the usual symptoms of the neurosis connected with a deficiency are tenseness, depression, and increased sensitivity. It is known that adequate nutrition is closely related to the ability of a person to think constructively. It is also known that poor nutrition can cause mental illness and even suicidal tendencies. For example, an absence of niacinamide in the diet can produce strong psychotic symptoms. The supplying of this vitamin has opened the doors of freedom to many mentally sick people.

Even the so-called natural breakdown in old people can now be slowed down and their mental faculties kept bright and alert, if their nutrition is ample and well-balanced, according to Dr Max Millman writing in *Today's Health*. Some clear-cut cases of mental illness can now be traced to nutritional deficiencies. A study of the effect of food on man's mind is throwing a bright light upon the undeniable fact that his mind and body are two manifestations of the same thing, so that what affects one must also affect the other.

Refined Sugar and Nerves

Refined sugar is a food from which man has removed all the valuable B-complex vitamins and minerals to leave a white residue which gives rise to acidity in the body and irritability in the mind. Dr Victor Lorenc, in the French health magazine *La Vie Claire*, wrote a series of articles on 'white sugar and its effect upon the body'. He showed that white sugar causes nervous irritation. It is so refined that all that is left is a dead acid; sweetnesss without sustenance. One of the white sugar's worst features, as we have seen, is that it immobilizes calcium.

Man's Fight Against Pain

The various types of nervous disorders cause people to turn to pain-killers such as paracetamol and aspirin products for relief. There are dozens of such products on the market under different names, but they mostly consist of three or four drugs—acetylsalicylic acid, paracetamol, and caffeine or codeine—all drugs, all pain-killers, but not one of them pain-curers. So great is the demand for these pain-killers that they are sold in general grocery shops and supermarkets as well as in chemists' shops.

But what is the unhappy sequel to this universal form of drug addiction? To get the same pain-killing result you have to constantly increase the dose. The more you increase the dose, the more you are poisoning your entire system. The more you poison your system, the more chronic and the more intense the pains become. And so the vicious circle goes round and round, with the victim getting worse and worse. One reason he gets worse is that these drugs often leach the vitamins out of his system, and before long his general health declines.

What is the Answer?

The logical answer to any form of nerve trouble is twofold. First, remove the causes of the nerve trouble. Second, make good the deficiencies of the vital factors so necessary to sound nerve health.

Gayelord Hauser (who died recently at the grand age of 89 years) created a new health era in America, with his researches, writings and lectures. He writes of the importance, first, of the vitamin B deficiency as a cause of nervous disorders: 'How much do you think it would be worth for you to know of a substance, easily available, which would increase your appetite, help digestion, protect you against nervous disorders, assure you freedom from constipation and generally promote your well-being? A hundred dollars? A thousand? Well, you have this knowledge for nothing. This substance is vitamin B complex, a powerful element present in many of the foods you are eating this very day. It can do all the things I mentioned—and more.' The B-complex vitamins strengthen the nerves, help to prevent constipation and make for calmness and balance.

A Convincing Test

Before very much was known about nutrition, medical science considered that nervous disorders arose largely from the tempo of living; from noise, stress and strain upon the nervous system. These are factors of course, but they are by no means so important as nutrition, particularly in B-complex vitamins.

Gayelord Hauser tells of two scientists of the University of Chicago, Drs E. R. Balken and S. Maurer, who with the co-operation of the Chicago Education Board, conducted an experiment a few years ago on forty-six growing schoolchildren to determine the relationship between B-complex vitamins and brain activity. The children came from underprivileged homes whose diets included starchy food with some meat, but lacked milk, vegetables and fruit. This diet is deficient in B-complex vitamins. The children were between 5½ and 9 years old. Five were in the upper kindergarten, and forty-one were in the first grade.

The scientists controlled the children's lunches and during the first four weeks no additional B-complex vitamins were given. From the fifth week and continuing through the twentieth week, 10g (about ⅓ ounce) of food containing vitamin B-complex was included each day. Before the experiment began and at regular intervals thereafter, every child was given intelligence tests. When the trial period concluded, it revealed conclusively that each child had improved physically, while in mental exercises they were much brighter and less fidgety and nervous.

Pain Relief

An eminent American physician, Dr Tilden, states that he prefers not to use morphine and other pain-killing drugs for pain relief. He says: 'If my patient is suffering greatly when I am first called, I order him to be put into a hot bath and kept there until completely relieved and relaxed. The hot bath brings a comfort that does no harm. Morphine and other drugs check secretions and excretions and this is exactly what should not be done for nature is in the throes of a desperate effort at throwing off poison, and when the medical man stops this effort he is committing a crime against the re-establishment of health.'

Breakfast Foods and Polished Rice

If 'civilized' man doesn't refine wheat, he blows it out with steam into wheat flakes and 'bubbles', and toasts it in an oven to produce an allegedly attractive breakfast food, but after the high steam pressure and the toasting, its vitamin content and most of its food value has been destroyed. 'Most processed cereals contain almost no protein', according to Adelle Davis in *Let's Eat Right to Keep Fit* (published under Signet Books, by The New American Library Inc., 1633 Broadway, New York, New York 10019, USA, 1970). The author states that 'rice flakes and puffed wheat supply only one gramme of poor-quality protein per cup. Prepared cereals are largely pure starch.' Pure starch is devoid of vitamins, as well as protein. Man in his ignorance 'polishes' rice—a process that removes the husk and the valuable germ cell, leaving only a filling devitalized product. So we see how the people of the world have been systematically starved of the vital elements necessary for their health in general and for their nerves in particular. It is generally agreed by nutritional scientists that the chief and basic cause of this great crop of nervous disorders is the progressive removal of the food elements required for a healthy nervous system, and for the calm, self-possession that goes with it.

Degrees of Nerve Trouble

Nerve troubles take various forms, as we have seen, and they assume various degrees of seriousness. Most people suffer from slight nervous disorders all their lives. A relatively small percentage of people enjoy nerve calm, composure, poise, equability, self-possession under stress, and show an imperturbable quality to irritation. These are indeed the fortunate few. It is said that man does not appreciate the value of personal freedom until he has lost it, and the same may be said of a healthy nervous system. We take it for granted while we have it, and only value it when we've lost it.

What Experiments Reveal

There is a school of thought, still generally subscribed to by the average medical practitioner, which holds the view that nerve troubles are purely psychological. That is to say, they believe that nervous disorders are caused by worry and that the mind only is affected, and through the mind, the nervous system. Advanced medical science no longer subscribes to this theory. Laboratory experiments carried out with rats have produced remarkably interesting results, so far as nerves are concerned.

Any group of rats completely starved of B-complex vitamins quickly become irritable, jumpy and fightable. They lose their hair, break out in sores and eventually die. Autopsies held on these rats showed that the main nerve sheaths were highly inflamed. Where a group of rats were only partially starved the degeneration in their health was not so serious, but there was unmistakable evidence of irritability and quarrelsomeness. In contrast, other groups of rats fed with all the required elements for health, and especially the B-complex vitamins, showed no irritability, played happily, and lived healthily much beyond the normal lifespan. Autopsies on this group showed that the nerve sheaths were quite free from inflammation.

High Incidence of Nervous Disorders

No such laboratory experiments have been conducted with human beings, but medical science has abundant evidence that the high incidence of nervous disorders to which all civilized races are subject today is due chiefly to a vitamin B-complex deficiency in the diet of most men, women and children. Autopsies upon humans who have died of disease invariably show acute inflammation of the nerve sheaths.

Nutritional science subscribes to the opinion that the person whose diet is nutritionally sound, and rich in essential vitamins and minerals, is generally able to stand up to the rigorous demands of modern life and go about his daily tasks and bear with the worries and vexations of today with a remarkable degree of equanimity. It is no exaggeration to say that in a more rational era, when the science of nutrition is given pride of place in the lives of the people from birth to death, nervous disorders and all the terrors they give rise to (including unfortunate inmates of mental hospitals) will be a rare phenomenon.

Ten Corrective Principles

In the light of the foregoing evidence, we are now able to sum up the whole matter, and set forth the ten curative principles for nervous disorders of all kinds.

1. Cut out all the dead and devitalized foods from your diet: These include white bread, sugar, cakes, pastry, processed and packeted breakfast flakes, 'instant' foods, jams, confectionery, pickled foods, macaroni, spaghetti, condiments, soft drinks, jellies, and biscuits. All these foods are deficient in B-complex vitamins and calcium, essential for sound nerves.
2. Add to your diet all the foods rich in these very essentials,

such as wholemeal bread, wholemeal porridge grains, wheatgerm, brewer's yeast, molasses, milk, powdered skim-milk, cheese, and eggs.

3. A consistent effort should be made to supply the vitamins and minerals in which you are deficient. Take one 10mg vitamin B_1 tablet, two B-complex tablets and two calcium tablets (white), before each meal and before retiring. In addition, it is advisable to take the following mixture twice daily for its high calcium, phosphorus, vitamin B, lactose and protein content: one heaped dessertspoonful of powdered brewer's yeast, mixed with one heaped dessertspoonful of powdered skim-milk, in a tumbler of water. A spoonful of honey (thinned with hot water) can be added as a sweetening agent, if desired. This is a palatable and nourishing drink. Continue this practice until your nerves are back to normal, and then reduce the vitamin dosage by half.

4. Stop taking drug tablets or powders, such as aspirin and paracetamol. They deaden pain and relax the nerves temporarily, but in the long term they make the nervous system worse.

5. The B-complex vitamins, and foods rich in calcium, phosphorus, and protein, are the greatest nerve foods money can buy. They help to restore not only the nerves, but the health in general.

6. It is most important for good nerves that you cut out sugar, sweets, jam, soft drinks, and all white flour foods, as these dead carbohydrate foods neutralize the calcium in your blood stream. Substitute needed calcium. Honey contains both vitamins and minerals.

7. Phosphorus is also important for good nerves. It occurs in the body in association with calcium and the B-

complex. Phosphorus is an essential part of every cell
of which the body and brain is made. Fortunately,
phosphorus is generously distributed in foods, especially
in wholemeal, unrefined grains, liver, milk (in all its
forms) and wheatgerm. But whilst phosphorus is one
of the most generously supplied minerals in nature, we
can still suffer from a deficiency of it. Adelle Davis
describes how the deficiency comes about in *Vitality
Through Planned Nutrition*.

> From 70 to 80 per cent of the phosphorus used by the
> body is used in combination with calcium. If too little
> calcium is eaten to allow this combination to take place
> efficiently, then the phosphorus is excreted by the kidneys.
> Since phosphorus is largely excreted in the form of
> calcium-phosphorus salts, the body not only loses
> phosphorus but the much-needed calcium as well.

The main point to note is that, if phosphorus is to be
retained in the body, calcium must be generously
supplied in the diet. Vitamin D is also needed, to enable
the body to utilize its calcium and phosphorus
requirements.

8. Good nerves need ample sleep, rest and relaxation. Sleep
can best be wooed by tiredness through normal activities,
but not by burning up one's vitality in unhealthy
excitements. Adequate calcium and B-complex vitamins
are essential to sound sleep. If you have been working
late at some mental task, sleep is best induced by a bath
and a rub down, or by exercise, which are both designed
to draw the blood away from the brain.

9. A sound nervous organization is the outcome of sound
health, and good general tone of mind and body.
Cultivate the art of relaxing at every opportunity.

Periodically through the day examine yourself for tenseness—tense muscles, tense expression, tense thoughts—and relax. Relaxation is a gift of the gods. Cultivate it!

10. Cultivate a philosophic mental attitude. You're not the only one with troubles, and worry by itself never solved anything. And remember this: the worries of today are forgotten tomorrow. Can you recall what you were worrying about this time last year? Or this time last month? I doubt it. If you are a natural worrier, you will find yourself worrying less and less as your health improves. The right mental attitude and a little philosophy, are both helpful factors in restoring the nervous organization to normal. Experience shows that anyone who consistently applies the foregoing principles for a few months will master the worst types of nervous disorder.

The Hunzas

Although the studies and observations referred to below took place some sixty or more years ago, the principles laid down apply even more today. They refer to a people called the Hunzas, and though most of us cannot emulate the lifestyles of these people, there is no reason why we should not learn from them and attempt at least some of their philosophies upon ourselves.

Dr Sir Robert McCarrison, C.I.E., M.D., D.Sc., LL.D., F.R.C.P., one time physician to the Viceroy of India, and an eminent nutritional scientist, gave the following report on the Hunzas, who follow the principles of sound nutrition with amazing results.

The Hunzas live in the north of India, and Dr McCarrison

describes their magnificent physical condition:

> The diet of these people corresponds in many ways to that of the Sikhs, but they eat less meat, and, their stock being limited to goats, their consumption of milk and milk products is less than that of the Sikhs. But they are great fruit-eaters, especially of apricots and mulberries, which they use in both the raw and the sun-dried state. The power of endurance of these people is extraordinary: to see a man of this race throw off his scanty garments, revealing a figure which would delight the eye of a Rodin, and plunge into a glacier-fed river in the middle of winter, with as much unconcern as many of us would take a tepid bath, is to realize that perfection of physique and great physical endurance are attainable on the simplest of foods, provided these be of the right kind.
>
> These people are long-lived and vigorous in old age. Among them the ailments too common in our own people—such as gastro-intestinal disorders, colitis, gastric and duodenal ulcer and cancer—are extraordinarily uncommon, and I have no doubt whatever in my own mind that their freedom from these scourges of modern civilization is due to three things: (1) their use of simple, natural foodstuffs of the right kind; (2) their vigorous outdoor life, and (3) their fine bracing climate. It is some years since I drew attention to the freedom of these people from any of the maladies which so commonly afflict our own people, and found a reason for it in their use of simple foodstuffs. . . With the Hunzas, resistance to infection is remarkable. . . Cancer is so rare that in nine years's practice I never came across a single case of it.

Sir Robert McCarrison was impressed, as other observers had been before him, with the striking contrast between the manly, stalwart and resolute races in Northern India, and the poorly developed, toneless and supine peoples of Southern India. He found that the diet of the people who lived around Madras, the worst diet in all India, was based on rice which has been soaked and polished, thus removing most of the vitamins and minerals. The Madrasi take little milk, little fruit or vegetables, drink coffee with sugar, and chew the betel nut. Their diet was deficient in vitamins, minerals and flesh-building proteins, and it was rare for anyone to live beyond forty.

Comment on the McCarrison Report

In *Health via Food*, Dr Howard Hay makes the following commentary on the report of Sir Robert McCarrison:

> Numerous instances of longevity are reported from various quarters proving that men can, under certain circumstances, live to a much greater age than the usual span. Perhaps the most striking instance in recent times is furnished by Dr Sir Robert McCarrison, formerly of the British Army Medical Service, who reports that in a colony in the Himalayan region he found natives who were so old that it would be hard to believe their records correct, yet he was not able to detect possible errors in the way of keeping these records. Ages up to and well beyond a century were very common among them. He found men of well attested age up to 100 years and over recently married and raising families of healthy children. Men said to be well over 100 years of age were working in the fields with younger men and doing as much work as any, in fact, looking so like the younger men that he was not able to distinguish the older from the younger.
>
> Beyond a small amount of milk or cheese, which were considered luxuries, the rest of the food consisted of grains in their normal state, nuts, vegetables and fruits and most of this was eaten raw. He reported that these people were never sick; they had none of the usual diseases of the civilized countries. They could not afford to cause them. There was,

during his nine years' residence in this post, no case of indigestion, constipation, appendicitis, gastric or duodenal ulcer; no cancer, tuberculosis, kidney disease, gallstones, asthma, hay fever; he never heard of a case of cold or pneumonia or pleurisy. Is it possible that these people live so long and are so free from disease because they live very largely on the natural foods?. . . The largest mass example of longevity is that furnished by Sir Robert McCarrison, and surely comprises enough instances to make a sort of criterion that favours natural foods.

What McCarrison Did

Writing in his book, *The Wheel of Health*, Dr G. T. Wrench states:

Robert McCarrison, now Major-General Sir Robert McCarrison, qualified as a medical practitioner at Queen's University, Belfast in 1900. He entered the Indian Medical Service and sailed for India on his twenty-third birthday. He was posted as regimental medical officer to the Indian troops, stationed as warden to the frontier march of Chitral, between the Gilgit Agency on the East and Afghanistan on the West, in the heart of a country likely to prove one of utmost significance in the history of food. McCarrison had the inborn mind of a research worker. He quickly displayed it in the accustomed manner of medical research. In 1913 he was transferred to the Central Institute, Kasauli, with all that its well equipped laboratories, scientific colleagues and literature offered.

In 1927 McCarrison was appointed Director of Nutrition Research in India under the research Fund Association. He was not only director, he was, as he told the members of the Royal Commission on Agriculture in India, the only officer engaged on work on nutrition, so he had, as it were, only to direct himself. He was given a laboratory and headquarters at Coonoor, upon the beautiful Nilgira plateau of the Madras Presidency, and there he directed his work and that of his excellent Indian assistants to the transference of the health of the Hunza, Sikh and Pathan to experimental science.

For this work McCarrison chose albino rats. Rats are largely used in nutritional laboratories. They offer many advantages for experimental work on foods. They are omnivorous and they like practically all human food. They are small animals and therefore cheap to feed. They breed readily in captivity, and their span of life is short, so that their whole life history can be watched. The first object of McCarrison was to see if the rats in their small sphere of life could be made exceptional in physique and health. He put them in good conditions of air, sunlight and cleanliness, and he chose as a diet for them, one based on those of the three people of excellent physique, the Hunza, the Pathans and the Sikhs.

Disease was Abolished!

The diet given to the rats was chapattis, a flat bread made of wholemeal wheat flour, lightly smeared with fresh butter, sprouted pulse, fresh raw carrots, and fresh raw cabbage libitum, unboiled milk, a small ration of meat with bones once a week and an abundance of water, both the drinking and washing. In this experiment 1189 rats were watched from birth to the twenty-seventh month, an age in the rat which corresponds to that of about fifty-five years in a man. The rats were killed and carefully examined at all ages up to the twenty-seventh month of life by naked-eye post-mortem examination. The result was very remarkable. Disease was abolished. This astonishing consequence, however, must be given in McCarrison's own words in the first of two lectures given at the College of Surgeons in 1931.

'During the past two and a quarter years there has been no case of illness in the "universe" of albino rats, no death from natural causes in the adult stock, and, but for a few accidental deaths, no infantile mortality. Both clinically and at post-mortem examination this stock has been shown to be remarkably free from disease. It may be that some of them have cryptic disease of one kind or another, but, if so I have failed to find either clinical or microscopical evidence of it.'

By putting the rats on a diet similar to that of certain people of northern India the rats became 'hunzarised', that is they 'enjoyed remarkable freedom from disease', words used by McCarrison in 1925 of the Hunza. They even went further. Except for an occasional tapeworm cyst they had no visible disease at all.

Diet, the Key to Health

The only thing, therefore, that was common to rat and man in this first experiment was the diet. Here in the great clefts of Hunza was a little oasis of a few thousand beings of almost perfect health, and here in the cages of Coonoor was a little oasis of a thousand or more albino rats in perfect health. The only link connection between these two otherwise dissimilar sets of living things was a similar kind of diet.

McCarrison now linked up other batches of rats in the same constant conditions of cleanliness and comfort with other peoples of India by the diets. He was in a most enviable position for trying out diets as a whole. The Indian sub-continent provides so many different races and different habits and diets. Hence McCarrison was able to sit in his sanctum at Coonoor and connect up his rats with teeming peoples near and far, and in the mirror of the rats read the dietetic fates of the peoples of Bengal and Madras, consisting of rice, pulses, vegetables, condiments, perhaps a little milk. He gave these to rats.

Now this diet immediately opened the lid of Pandora's box

for the rats of Coonoor, and diseases and miseries of many kinds flew forth. McCarrison made a list of them as found by him in 2243 rats fed on faulty Indian diets. The rats which were fed on the diets eaten by millions of Indians of Bengal and Madras, got diseases of every organ they possessed, namely, eyes, noses, ears, lungs, hearts, stomachs, intestines, kidneys, bladders, reproductive organs, blood, ordinary glands, special glands and nerves. The liver and brain, it may be noted, do not occur in the list. The liver was in fact found to be diseased in conjunction with the diseases of the gastro-intestinal tract. The examination of the brain requires a careful opening of the small bony brain case of the rat and adds greatly to the time needed for post-mortem examinations. In a list given five years later in the Cantor Lectures, McCarrison adds a few further diseases such as general weakness, lassitude, irritability, loss of hair, ulcers, boils, bad breath, crooked spines, distorted vertebrae, and so on.

Index